Diabetes U̶n̶p̶a̶c̶k̶e̶d

Just Science and Sense
No Sugar Coating

Various Authors
In support of The Noakes Foundation

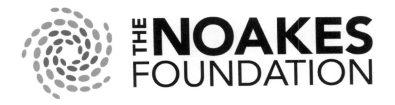

Published by Columbus Publishing Ltd 2017

www.columbuspublishing.co.uk

ISBN 978-1-907797-58-3

Rev 20170620

Edited by Dr Zoë Harcombe

Cover design by Lewis Kokoc

Typesetting by Raffaele Bolelli Gallevi

Thank you to Scott Murdoch, for giving his permission to use his iconic 'Tokyo subway' image on page 61.

COLUMBUS PUBLISHING

Acknowledgements and Dedication

Acknowledgements

We would like to thank all the authors of this book, who have kindly shared their research and wisdom freely, so that anyone with diabetes, or an interest in diabetes, may understand that official advice may not be good advice. We particularly thank the authors for generously donating their work, so that The Noakes Foundation will benefit as a result of this publication.

This book would not be what it is without the valued real-life stories shared by Indya, Lindy, Neil and Nigel and to Gareth Dupre, who so expertly and sensitively helped them to write their stories.

We would also like to thank Peggy Matthews and Raffaele Bolelli Gallevi for their meticulous review of the manuscript.

Dedication

This book is dedicated to all diabetics, to everyone who knows a diabetic and to anyone who could become diabetic. It is a travesty that we have been advised to: "Base meals on starchy foods." There is another way.

Contents

About The Noakes Foundation

My interest in diabetes – and the many other names it has – is deeply personal. It's personal to me and to my country. South Africa is the third most obese nation in the world – a figure that constantly befuddles me. We are a country with an enormous land mass and sufficient space and agri-diversity to sufficiently feed our country and flourish. We have a concentration of many world leading brains, bodies, minds, athletes and a country that has no reason to be suffering from diseases of the first world. What went wrong and why here?

The biggest injustice we have seen to date, at The Noakes Foundation and "Eat Better South Africa!", has been the hard truth that the poorest seem to get the sickest and most overweight first. This is not only the case with diabetes, but its underlying early flag, insulin resistance and the various other diseases that we now know are associated with it. I was sketchily diagnosed with insulin resistance at the age of 21 and now know that this disease drives various other illnesses: hypertension, heart disease, obesity, inflammation, arthritis, gout, dementia, Alzheimer's and possibly even many metabolic cancers.

There are lists of thousands, if not hundreds of thousands, of people who have suffered through years and decades of incorrect dietary management of a chronic condition. This list keeps growing and, as we gather the endless evidence of self-reported disease remission or reversal due to ketogenic or LCHF transition, we are blown away daily by how many forms of malaise are rectified by this most simple information.

It is information that does not rely on expensive drugs or massive medical intervention. Anyone who has suffered, or is still suffering from this syndrome, which affects pretty much everything in the human body – anyone who has struggled with prediabetes or diabetes knows this. Within weeks something massive changes metabolically and you are given another chance at vitality.

For me, I felt like I had my life back and my humanity and brain restored, after decades of following the wrong advice that had gotten me ill in the first place.

At The Noakes Foundation, we raise funds to support research, but also to support the approximately 46.5 million South Africans who are not on private medical aid and are thus not able to get the world class care that less than 18 percent of our country affords in the privatised system. It is these people who are worst off; with little or no support and insufficient regular medical advice, diabetes is an ever-growing burden and dynamite that has now taken over HIV deaths in our country. It is a bomb that has already gone off. There is not a second to waste to make the change, cut the sugars and to start asking why we got here and how we can fix things for future generations. Many people need to wake up, even the ones who are not diabetic or sick and are managing on the current diet, but still feeding their children endless refined carbs and sugars and thinking *'it won't happen to us'*.

A while ago, a top medical insurance leader who had initially been vehemently against the Banting movement in South Africa and outspoken against the approach Prof Noakes was taking to diabetes management, came to meet us to apologise. Just after he had left this influential role, which had set up our largest private medical aid in a way that denied LCHF eating and even penalised its members for eating this way (and still does today), his daughter had been diagnosed as a Type 1 diabetic. Overnight, he and his wife had changed their kitchen and got the whole family Banting. Their daughter is now controlling her diabetes without insulin and all their other children are off ADD medication. They will never go back. He said he would never have imagined how his perfectly healthy child could get this condition and now that his eyes are opened, they will never go back.

We don't want children needing insulin before parents wake up. Change needs to happen before children reach that stage. Long before. They need simple information to understand the exaggerated amounts of toxic sugars and insulin spinning carbs that are hidden in their children's average foods.

It is more critical now to our nation's survival than anything else. Our primary concern needs to be to sort out the millions of children in South Africa who are living on more than 80 percent maize and refined wheat-based products in their diets.

Children are getting bottles filled with sugar-filled fizzy drinks instead of water or milk and then graduating onto school meals of maize (known as pap here) and a soft drink. One school meal programme, which we want to fund, currently relies on yesterday's bread rolls from local supermarkets to make slop soup for 86,000 children. For these children it is their only meal of the day.

The reality here is simple and visible. Everyone is getting fatter and sicker at the same time. It's the same as malnourishment, presenting itself in a bigger costume. Schools are desperate. The navy is struggling with uniform sizes and basic fitness levels. The time bomb is ticking.

It is not dissimilar to what is happening in the USA and the UK. While South Africans in townships are feeding their children pap at under 10 USD cents a meal, Americans are seemingly obliviously handing over Pop Tarts for breakfast, as if they are a healthy start to the day.

Diabesity as we call it and its effects may be the single most uniting factor of humanity. It is undiscerning and speaks one sugar-fuelled common language as we see the Far East being the last but equally fast hit.

The truth of this situation is so dire that in order to effect change, we need help from everyone: the academics and scientists and their extraordinary minds and problem-solving abilities; the doctors and specialists who are on the ground addressing the daily realities of chronic disease and fighting up-hill battles; the nurses and dieticians. Mostly, it's going to take every single person to change things, cut the sugar and carbs and generate industry demand to change. It's going to take every mother's purse, both in South Africa and the world, to change the situation from the bottom up.

The team here in Cape Town and I would like to offer our heartfelt thanks to each of the incredible, passionate authors and contributors to this book for offering their royalties to The Noakes Foundation and Eat Better South Africa!

We would also like to thank the formidable Harcombes for their depth of vision and the work they do in the world for this great offering and idea!

We have committed to two years of making our country and then the world a better place with our simple and profound educational programmes in informal settlements. Royalties of this book will all go to Eat Better South Africa and you can find us on Facebook or on our website to hear what we are up to, to get in touch or find out about how you can help become a part of the answers we know and understand to work.

We would like to invite you to engage, contribute, buy better and also to speak up and challenge what is.

Today is the day!

Jayne Bullen

COO @ The Noakes Foundation
www.thenoakesfoundation.org

About The Noakes Foundation

The Noakes Foundation was founded in 2012 by Professor Tim Noakes. It was established in response to the critical need for robust research into nutrition. The Foundation is a Non-Profit Organisation founded for public benefit which aims to advance medical science's understanding of the benefits of a low-carbohydrate healthy high fat (LCHF) diet by providing evidence-based information on optimum nutrition. The Foundation's key goal is to change the way South Africa, and hopefully the world, thinks about food and nutrition. The obesity and Type 2 diabetes epidemics are set to cripple global health care within the next 10 years, something needs to be done before this happens. The Noakes Foundation is taking action.

Eat Better South Africa!

The Noakes Foundation soon realised that the poorest communities around South Africa, whose diets mainly consist of maize and maize products, were unaware of the dangers of excessive sugar and carbohydrate consumption. This has resulted in an unprecedented increase in cases of obesity, Type 2 diabetes, and other metabolic syndromes. Thus the Noakes Foundation team established Eat Better South Africa! (EBSA)- the community outreach branch of The Noakes Foundation. EBSA is a programme aimed at educating people from lower income areas, teaching them to get better by eating better. Men and women from these communities sign up to a six-week course where they learn about the benefits of a low carb high healthy fat diet and are assisted in making better food choices through nutritional education, meal and budget planning, and general nutritional awareness.

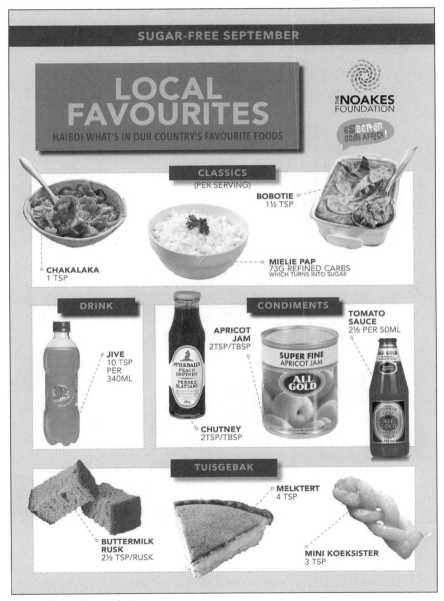

Educational Material

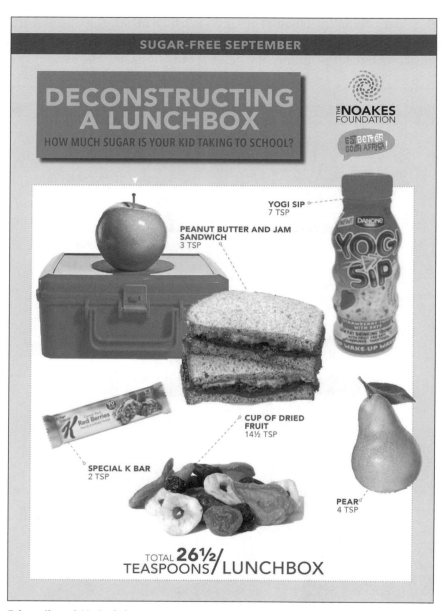

DECONSTRUCTING A LUNCHBOX
HOW MUCH SUGAR IS YOUR KID TAKING TO SCHOOL?

THE NOAKES FOUNDATION

Eat Better SOUTH AFRICA!

YOGI SIP
7 TSP

PEANUT BUTTER AND JAM SANDWICH
3 TSP

CUP OF DRIED FRUIT
14½ TSP

SPECIAL K BAR
2 TSP

PEAR
4 TSP

TOTAL **26½** TEASPOONS / LUNCHBOX

Educational Material

A DIETICIAN'S MEAL PLAN FOR DIABETES

THE GOAL OF DIABETES MANAGEMENT IS TO STABILIZE BLOOD GLUCOSE LEVELS AND KEEP IT WITHIN THE NORMAL LOW RANGE:

CARBOHYDRATES
are broken down into glucose in the body - carbs have the most significant impact on blood sugar-they cause it to spike significantly.

PROTEINS
are broken down into amino acids which are needed for growth and repair of the body. When consumed alone, protein does not generate a rise in blood sugar levels.

FATS
are broken down into triglycerides which are used for energy and a variety of other functions within the body, for example hormone production and for keeping cell membranes healthy. Like protein, fat has significantly less impact on blood sugar than carbo-hydrates. When consumed alone, ingested fats have little to no bearing on blood sugar levels.

A DIETICIANS DIABETIC MEAL PLAN DECONSTRUCTED:

THE NOAKES FOUNDATION

This meal plan is very high in carbs and sugars, 34 tsps of added sugars per day will have a drastic effect on a diabetics blood sugar levels. Protein and fat have little to no effect on blood sugar levels, this is why The Noakes Foundation recommends a low carb high fat diet for diabetics.

MEAL	CARB CONTENT	SUGAR CONTENT
BREAKFAST		
Muesli & low-fat milk	66g	26g
Banana & date muffin	57g	21g
Tea / coffee with low-fat milk	2g	2g
SNACK		
Peanuts & raisins	15g	12g
Tea / coffee with low-fat milk	2g	2g
LUNCH		
Steak	0g	0g
Corn on the cob with margarine	14g	2g
Salad	2g	0g
Pear	25g	16g
Low-fat yogurt	31g	5g
Tea / coffee with low-fat milk	2g	2g
SNACK		
Dried apricots	4g	4g
Tea / coffee with low-fat milk	2g	2g
DINNER		
Lean tomato mince	4g	2g
Pasta	42g	0g
Mixed vegetables	9g	2g
Apple & cabbage salad with low-fat dressing	15g	10g
Sliced plums with artificial sweetener	7g	6g
Tea / coffee with low-fat milk	2g	2g
SNACK	7g	1g
Crackers with margarine	21g	20g
Milo & low-fat milk		
TOTAL	**329g**	**137 grams = 34 tsp of sugar**

A Meal Plan prescribed by a Dietitian

Introduction

By Dr Zoë Harcombe, Ph.D

My teenage brother, Adrian, had been in Canada at a scouting convention for three weeks. When we waved him off he had been in great shape – a natural sportsman excelling at all games, but cricket, hockey and swimming especially. A week into his trip, our relatives in Toronto contacted us to say that Adrian had left the event 'suffering exhaustion' and was staying with them, but they were quite worried about his weight loss. When we collected Adrian from the airport, he was a shadow of the young man we had seen not even a month earlier.

A mad cricket fan, Adrian installed himself in front of the TV when he got home – watching every ball of five day matches, as he loved to do. It was the summer holidays, so we had much freedom to spend our days. I would do anything for my big brother so when he gave me some coins, and asked me to pop to the local shop to get some fizzy pop, I happily set off on my bike. No sooner had I delivered a two-litre bottle, Adrian would be asking me to take the previous bottle back for the deposit and to get another one. His thirst was insatiable.

I returned from one such fizzy drink excursion to a note from mum saying that she'd decided to take Adrian to hospital. Later that afternoon, dad came home early from work, collected me and we headed off to the hospital together. Adrian was already in a hospital bed with mum on one side and a consultant on the other. The endocrinologist gave the whole family a serious talk about what life would be like, now that we were living with a Type 1 diabetic.

The symptoms were so obvious – dramatic weight loss and insatiable thirst – that Adrian should have been diagnosed in Canada. But this was long before the current era of diabetes awareness. We were shocked and the messages delivered with gravity by the consultant stuck with me from that day. We were taught how to recognise low blood glucose (too much insulin) and high blood glucose (too much sugar). If experiencing hypoglycemia (low blood glucose), Adrian would likely become withdrawn, dopey, maybe a bit incoherent. His hands might shake and he might feel clammy to the touch. If experiencing hyperglycemia (high blood glucose), Adrian might appear drunk, gregarious, 'high' – he was given a bracelet announcing that he was a Type 1 Diabetic, so that he wouldn't be mistaken for a drunk if a hyper-episode occurred.

Family members were trained to administer an insulin injection and we kept sugar cubes to hand, so that we could counter 'a hypo' as necessary. I used to help Adrian to inject in the arm, as he could more easily inject himself in the leg and this avoided particular skin areas becoming over-used.

This was my introduction to diabetes – Type 1 Diabetes Mellitus (T1DM) specifically – the rarer kind. The one that we still don't fully understand. Is it hereditary? Is it an auto-immune condition? Why do some people get it and not others? Why did it only used to occur in young people and yet we now have middle aged people being diagnosed with T1DM? The type, which represents fewer than 10% of all cases of diabetes is a complex condition indeed.

In contrast, Type 2 Diabetes Mellitus (T2DM) is emerging as the condition that is easier to understand and certainly the one that is easier to address. It is by far the more common type (more than 90% of diabetes cases) and one that is now being described as an epidemic. Why? Why has T2DM gone from being "what granny with a sweet tooth gets" to a condition seen in children?

The beliefs we share

This book is a collection of chapters by thought leaders, academics and doctors with personal and/or patient experience of diabetes – mostly T2DM, by virtue of the proportion of diabetes that this type comprises. The traditional view of diabetes is that it is a "chronic and progressive" condition and that nothing can be done about it. Serious complications include loss of eyesight, amputations and death. The writers in this book approach diabetes from many different angles, but they all share one common belief: Diabetes does not need to be "chronic and progressive." Both types can be substantially alleviated and T2DM can be 'reversed'.

A quick word on words here, as the idea that T2DM can be 'reversed' or 'cured' is contentious. May I suggest that this comes down to more terminology and may I propose a clarification to ease the contention? I don't think that T2DM can be reversed *per se*, in that a person diagnosed with T2DM will have T2DM from that point on. However, it is clear that lifestyle changes can be made by someone with T2DM, enabling them to get to the point that they effectively don't have T2DM. The T2DM person can make changes such that they would not be diagnosed with T2DM today. To that extent, the T2DM has been reversed or cured. If the person resumed their previous lifestyle, the changes would abate and the T2DM would manifest itself again. Some people refer to T2DM being 'in remission' and I prefer this term, as it more accurately describes where the person is. However, I completely understand the importance of terminology in this world. I have met many people at conferences who introduce themselves by saying "I'm a cured Type 2 diabetic" or "I have reversed my diabetes." The idea that this 'chronic and progressive' disease can be 'reversed' is hugely motivational to people diagnosed with T2DM. If this means that the words 'reversed' and 'cured' are used in preference to 'in remission' – don't knock it. Anything that motivates individuals to dramatically improve their health is to be encouraged, not discouraged.

So what are these changes? How can T2DM be reversed? The writers in this book share the common belief that diabetes does not need to be chronic and progressive. We also share the common belief as to how. We know that the macronutrient that diabetics (both types) are least able to handle is carbohydrate. We therefore cannot understand that dietary advice for diabetics is to eat the majority of one's diet in the form of carbohydrate – the very substance that cannot be handled. (This is the same advice for non-diabetics, which is why we continue to make more people diabetic daily).

My husband, Andy, and I wanted to produce and publish a book, gathering together some of the finest minds worldwide, to give intelligent and interested readers some unconventional thinking on this serious condition. We want to stimulate thinking, share logic and personal/patient experiences and challenge the status quo that diabetics should "base their meals on starchy foods" and thus suffer the consequences of sugar ravages in their body as time goes by.

We have all donated our work for free and we are hoping that contributions from this book will raise valuable funds for The Noakes Foundation, founded by Professor Tim Noakes. This is particularly fitting for a number of reasons. First, the goal of The Noakes Foundation is "*To support the dietary revolution that will reverse the global epidemics of obesity and type 2 diabetes mellitus.*" This not-for profit organisation is thus perfectly suited to address the condition that this book is largely about. Second, Professor Noakes has been the inspiration to so many of us in this field. It is an honour for us to be working with the person who has been so evidence-led and determined to find the truth that he has ripped up one of his own early books! (The Lore of Running). Finally, Professor Noakes has been one of an elite few who have been put on trial, or worse – convicted with no trial – simply for daring to suggest that Type 2 diabetics should eat less carbohydrate.

The practitioners on trial

Jennifer Elliott

Jennifer Elliott had been a dietician for 35 years and for 10 of those had recommended carbohydrate restriction to clients with T2DM. She was taught the standard advice – a low-fat diet, with plenty of whole grains, fruit and vegetables. Her daughter developed a weight problem between the ages of 12 and 14 and had classic abdominal obesity. A general practitioner tested the young girl for insulin resistance and confirmed the diagnosis. Jennifer began her own research into insulin resistance and found a wealth of evidence that had not been taught in dietetics training. It became clear to Jennifer that carbohydrate was *not* the friend of diabetics and/or those with insulin resistance. Jennifer changed her daughter's diet and started to change the diet of clients similarly afflicted. The results were immediate: weight loss; improved blood glucose levels; and a reduced need for medications.

You would think that the dietetic association would have been thrilled and would have sought to emulate the advice that had proved so effective. The opposite happened. Jennifer was reported by a Dietitians Association of Australia (DAA) registered dietician and charged with using a "non-evidence-based" approach.

The Dietitians Association of Australia (DAA) conducted the investigations into the allegation. You can check the conflicts of the official body for dieticians in Australia for yourself. Around the time that Jennifer was under investigation, the "corporate partners" of the DAA included

Campbell Arnott's "one of the largest food manufacturers in Australia"; Nestle; and the Australian Breakfast Cereal Manufacturers Forum.

The outcome of the investigation was that Jennifer was de-registered by the DAA in May 2015. Her employer, a local Health District, dismissed her as a result.

Jennifer paid a heavy personal and financial price for suggesting that people who can't handle carbohydrate should eat less of it.

Gary Fettke

Australian dieticians have shown themselves to be particularly vicious in their determination to eliminate any practitioners stepping outside their own belief system. Surgeon Dr Gary Fettke was the next high profile health practitioner to be targeted by those wedded to the low fat high carb dietary advice. Gary is a surgeon. He amputates limbs. He mainly amputates the limbs of diabetics whose bodies have been damaged by the ravages of sugar. As a doctor, who took an oath to "first do no harm", he felt compelled to advise patients that – if they didn't consume the sugar that was destroying their limbs, he wouldn't need to cut their limbs off. That's the kind of direct guy that Gary is!

Again – you would think that this limb and life saving advice would be welcome. Again you'd be wrong. Again it was a dietician who (anonymously) reported Gary – this time the Australian Health Practitioners Regulatory Authority (AHPRA) acted as judge and jury. After two years, in August 2016, they ruled that Gary must not give nutritional advice to patients. Specifically they said: "In particular that he does not provide specific advice or recommendations on the subject of nutrition and how it relates to the management of diabetes or the treatment and/or prevention of cancer."

Have dieticians managed to silence these two pioneers? Has the DAA monopoly on low-fat diet advice been preserved? Thankfully not. As of early 2017, Gary has defied the authorities and gone back to speaking out publicly on nutrition and in particular the benefits of Low Carbohydrate Healthy Fat living. It's just too important for him. As he said: "Once you see the results for people, you cannot unsee them." Thanks to the networking wonder that is the internet, Jennifer's personal web site (babyboomersandbellies.com) prevails and she has partnered with Franziska Spritzler, a low carb dietician, to offer a program for diabetes.

Professor Tim Noakes

A different continent, but a similar story. Professor Tim Noakes had gained such a following in South Africa that the term "Banting"[1] had become commonplace. When I spoke at a conference in Cape Town in February 2015, there were two Banting restaurants and it was quite normal to see menu items tagged with "Banting" or "LCHF" (low carb high fat) to indicate their suitability for this way of eating.

On 3 February 2014, someone called Pippa Leenstra tweeted: *"@ProfTimNoakes @SalCreed is LCHF eating OK for breastfeeding mums? Worried about all the dairy + cauliflower = wind for babies??"* (@SalCreed is Sally-Ann Creed, a co-author of The Real Meal Revolution with Tim).

On 5 Feb 2014, Tim tweeted: *"@pippaleenstra @SalCreed Baby doesn't eat the dairy and cauliflower. Just very healthy high fat breast milk. Key is to ween baby onto LCHF."*

This became the most expensive tweet in the history of twitter! A South African dietician, Claire Julsing Strydom, reported Tim to the Health Professions Council of South Africa (HPCSA). Tim was charged with giving unconventional advice. Several million rand and three years later, the verdict was delivered on 21 April 2017. Tim was found not guilty of professional misconduct. In fact, the committee delivered verdicts on 10 aspects of the hearing and they found Tim not guilty for all 10 counts. However, 'the most expensive tweet' continues to accrue costs, as, at the time of this book going to print, the HPCSA had announced that it was going to appeal the decision.

Along with two other authors in this book (Dr Caryn Zinn and Nina Teicholz), I had the privilege of being invited by Tim to appear as an expert witness at the hearing, It was an extra-ordinary experience on so many levels: Extra-ordinary to present evidence and be cross-examined in an open court session in a foreign country; Extra-ordinary that something so monumental ostensibly started with a tweet[*]; Extra-ordinary that anyone could think that twitter is a doctors' surgery and that a doctor-patient relationship is even established with open exchanges; Extra-ordinary that one of the finest, A1 rated, scientists that South Africa will ever see has been

---

[*] During the hearing, it became clear that a particular paper had played a significant part in the prosecution of Professor Noakes. Several prosecution witnesses admitted to "waiting for" this particular paper so that they had the "evidence" to charge "the Prof."[2]

subjected to a witch-hunt for daring to point out that the dietary guidelines are not fit for purpose – for diabetics especially – if not, to avoid diabetes.

This case also involved one or more dieticians. The professional association for dieticians in South Africa is conflicted, as elsewhere. Russ Greene did an outstanding forensic on the conflicts of interest in the Professor Noakes hearing[3]. The common factors with Jennifer, Gary and Tim are dieticians protecting their non-evidence based, conventional thinking, with big food conflicts all over the crime scene. If John Grisham turned his attention to these cases, the book would need to appear in the non-fiction section.

Decent upstanding citizens should be utterly appalled that big food and dieticians are able to silence health practitioners who are simply trying to advise those who can't handle carbohydrate to cut back on it.

This book

It has been an honour for Andy and me to initiate, assemble and produce this book. I have had the privilege of editing it, which has enabled me to give you a taste of the delights you're in for...

Setting the scene

The scale of the problem is set out by Mike Gibbs, a Cambridge University graduate. Mike co-founded "OurPath" with Chris Edson, an Oxford University graduate. OurPath is an online education and behavioural change programme, which uses technology to address the growing burden of Type 2 diabetes. With a combination of dietary changes, exercise, support groups and other lifestyle interventions (better sleep and stress management, for example), Mike and Chris are trying to prevent people getting into the diabetes pipeline as well as helping those already living with T2DM to better manage the disease.

The rest of the section "Setting the scene" contains three chapters from three of the greatest thinkers in the world on diabetes. The genius of Dr Malcolm Kendrick, Dr Jason Fung and, perhaps less well known to some of you, Dr Robert Cywes, kicks off the book in brilliant and witty style. The way that these men think is simply delightful. It is concise, logical, memorable and so darned sensible that you read their contributions thinking – why, why, why do the powers-that-be not see this?

Malcolm sets out to explain what diabetes is, in as simple a way as possible, while cautioning that, as H. L. Mencken famously said "For every complex problem there is a solution that is simple, easy to understand – and wrong." Malcolm keeps it as simple and right as is possible. What is the slow progression of diabetes? Is it impaired glucose tolerance or impaired fasting tolerance? Do we have the right focus on sugar? insulin? Is what we observe insulin resistance, or are the liver and muscles simply full of glycogen causing a re-direction of glucose? How can lipodystrophy or PIMA Indians help with our thinking?

Jason asks similar questions – what is T2DM? What causes it? What's the difference between Type 1 and Type 2 in terms of insulin? Jason takes us through his insulin resistance model of diabetes. What causes insulin resistance? What is hyperinsulinemia? Why do we develop insulin resistance? Does it serve any useful purpose? With wonderful imagery and analogies – from suitcases to sugar bowls to Japanese subway pushers – Jason takes us on a tour-de-force to see what life is really like in 'DiabetesVille' ☺

I had the privilege of seeing Dr Robert Cywes present at the Feb 2015 conference in Cape Town, South Africa. A self-confessed carbohydrate addict (in remission!), Robert understands carbohydrate addiction better than anyone I have ever come across. He just gets it. He talks, as he writes, in sound bites. You feel like you want to write down what he's just said, because it's so insightful. While you're writing, the next thing he says is equally insightful and you want to write this down too. Then you realise that you want to write down everything he says because it's all equally quotable and brilliant. Here are some of my favourite quotations from his chapter: "Asking a diabetic to count their carbohydrates is no different than asking an alcoholic to count their drinks." "The cause of T2DM is not a lack of insulin, it is a chronic excess of carbohydrate consumption that results in genetically predetermined failure of the insulin-glucagon blood glucose management system."

Robert is a practising bariatric surgeon, but he tries to use very low carbohydrate diets as a preferable 'last resort' to bariatric surgery, which is usually called the last resort when very low carb diets have *not* been tried. If surgery is deemed necessary, Robert uses his knowledge of carbohydrate addiction to help him to help the patient after surgery. He knows that their stomach may have been taken away, but their addiction hasn't been surgically removed. As he says: "No operation on the stomach cures the head."

Our first case study in the book is Indya – one of Robert's patients and she credits him with saving her life. Just wait until you see her before and after pictures.

The different types

Section two opens with a Type 1 diabetic general practitioner from the UK, Dr Ian Lake, sharing how he transformed his own health after 20 years of following the conventional advice. He has stopped his progressive deterioration and he explains how – as well as giving invaluable information for any T1DMs keen to exercise and wondering how this can be done while managing their condition. Carbs, fats, background insulin and meal response insulin – all are wonderfully detailed in a chatty, first-person chapter, which gives a heartfelt insight into life as a T1DM.

Lars-Erik Litsfeldt is a T2DM from Scandinavia – part of the world known for leading the way with the low carbohydrate approach to obesity and diabetes. Lars shares his personal diagnosis as a T2DM and the traditional advice that he was given, alongside his discovery of a woman taking on the conventional world in Sweden – Dr Annika Dahlqvist. In November 2006, two dieticians reported Annika to the Swedish National Board of Health (sounds familiar?!) and I'll let Lars tell you what happened. I very much enjoyed the warmth and humour of Lars' chapter – some probably a result of a Swedish person incredibly writing for us in a foreign language. It's quite adorable in places.

Then we're back to the UK, honoured to have a contribution from the famous "Fixing Dad" team. Jen Whitington, has written an eloquent and moving chapter about her father-in-law, Geoff Whitington. Geoff's story has featured on BBC2 – one of the major UK television channels – and in the national press. Geoff and his son Anthony speak often at conferences and they have produced a book and a film of the family's inspirational and tear-jerking story.

Nigel is our next case study. Nigel was diagnosed with diabetes – the medical profession couldn't even decide which type he has. He discovered the low carb 'fix' for himself and, in six months, Nigel went from literally being at death's door, to being "fitter than he had been since a teenager." The response of his carb prescribing practitioners? Halving his HbA1c in such a short time was "too quick" and he should be more careful! He continued to ignore their advice.

The practitioners

Dr Caryn Zinn tells a page turner of a story about how her colleague, Professor Grant Schofield, made some 'outrageous' statements saying that low carb diets and saturated fat had been wrongly demonised. Caryn stormed off in search of the evidence 'to show him' and you'll have to read Chapter Eight to see what happened next. If I tell you that Caryn, like Gary, Jennifer and Tim above, became one of the practitioners at risk of being stopped from helping patients by zealous dieticians, you may be even more curious. My admiration for those within the system, who challenge the system, knows no bounds.

Dr Neville Wellington is on the board of The Noakes Foundation. He is also a doctor practising in Cape Town who was becoming increasingly upset at his inability to help the increasing number of T2DM people walking into his surgery. Neville was contacted by Professor Noakes in 2012. Tim shared with Neville his journey into evidence-based nutrition and how it led to low-carbohydrate diets, especially for diabetics. Neville followed along the same path and found the same. Neville now has quite a tool kit to help his patients and his chapter is an invaluable guide to glucose monitoring – why do it, when to do it, how to do it. "Ultimately, it becomes obvious that diabetes is controlled (or even reversed) one meal at a time." This is a wonderfully practical and helpful chapter for any diabetic and anyone who knows a diabetic – that's most of us. One of Neville's sentences should be pinned on fridges across the globe: "In general, it becomes very obvious that 'lows' (hypoglycemia) are caused by too much medication, and 'highs' (hyperglycemia) are caused by too much carbohydrate."

The final of our three practitioners is a GP (General Practitioner) in the UK. If you've seen Dr David Unwin present at conferences, you'll know he has a bedside manner to die for (no pun intended!) He is warm, calm and encouraging. David also currently has the excitement of a 5 year old on Christmas Eve because, like Caryn and Neville, he has – after 30 years as a GP – found something that works for his diabetic patients. He is getting the most extra-ordinary results – and these have not gone unnoticed. David was awarded the UK National NHS (National Health Service) Innovator of the Year award (2016) out of ten regional finalists.

Lindy's case study closes this section. Life took Lindy to Holland and, when she finally left the country, she had gained 40 kg and Type 2 diabetes. Faced with the usual advice of high carbohydrate intake and metformin, Lindy recalled having read one of my books and upped her reading – soon coming across Dr Jason Fung, Dr Andreas Eenfeldt and more. Lindy adopted a very low carbohydrate diet, embraced fat and you may be able to guess how that worked out.

The big issues

The final section is the big issues. You can read any of the book's chapters in any order you like and some of you may wish to start with these – or jump around from your favourite authors to new writers that you are keen to discover. In Chapter Eleven, I ask and answer the question: "Why do we eat so much carbohydrate?" There's a short answer (because we demonised fat), but the really interesting story is how, when and why we came to demonise fat. Thankfully that was the subject of my Ph.D, the finale of which I share in this chapter.

Dr Jeff Gerber and engineer Ivor Cummins pick up the baton of the diet-heart hypothesis and investigate why do diabetics die from heart disease? What a great question. There's a great answer too, as Jeff and Ivor walk us through atherosclerosis as a metabolic disease, the Framingham study and where cholesterol and insulin fit in with all of this. I loved this chapter. It should be compulsory to have doctors and engineers work together because the problem solving logic is just a joy to be swept away with. This is a first rate Irish-American collaboration.

The pièce de résistance comes from "The Prof", as he is affectionately known in the real food world – the professor among all professors: Professor Tim Noakes. Tim's chapter explains why low carbohydrate high fat (LCHF) diets are the only ethical option for people with diabetes (Tim focuses on T2DM, but T1DMs need to lower their carb intake to similar levels) and why virtually all athletes should also be adopting this way of eating. As you would expect from one of the world's few A1 rated scientists, this is an academic chapter, beautifully explained and well referenced. You will wonder at the end of it, as I did when I had the honour of being involved at his hearing, how is this man on trial for his advice? Why has he not been made head of public health in South Africa?!

We are thrilled to have the author of the best-selling, award-winning, "Big Fat Surprise" closing the book. That honour could have gone to Tim, but, as a huge fan of Nina's work himself, Tim will appreciate that this is the logical final chapter. When all the evidence has been presented – from thought leaders, surgeons, doctors, enlightened dieticians, academics, engineers and public health nutritionists – and all the evidence overwhelmingly concludes that carbohydrate is the worst macronutrient for diabetics, one is left baffled as to why governments have not already implemented change. Nina explains why – the interested parties, the money at stake, the conflicts embedded – there is no incentive to change from the perspective of big pharma or big food or the government bodies they lobby.

As Lars says in his chapter: "A moderately ill patient, with a long life, would be the perfect customer!"

Jason emailed me in the early stages of developing the book and, in his usual brilliant and concise way, he nailed it. What this book needs to show, he said is: 1) T2DM is reversible and 2) T2DM is a dietary disease, which demands a dietary solution. Drugs don't work.

I think we've done it – by gum, I really think we've done it.

Dr Zoë Harcombe, Ph.D

@zoeharcombe
zoeharcombe.com

Setting the scene

Chapter One

What is the scale of the problem?

Mike Gibbs

Diabetes is a global health epidemic. In a 2014 study, one of the biggest studies of its kind, scientists from Imperial College London reported that 422 million people worldwide were living with diabetes.[1] That's four times as many as in 1980, when 108 million people were living with the disease. That bears reiteration – the number of diabetics has quadrupled across the globe in just over 35 years.

Other studies have analysed the number of people likely to develop diabetes. The Centers for Disease Control and Prevention (CDC) reported that 86 million people were at risk in the United States in 2014.[2] That's an astounding one in three people.

As was mentioned in the introduction to this book, 'diabetes' is an umbrella term for a number of different subtypes of the disease. The most commonly talked about are Type 1 Diabetes Mellitus (T1DM) and Type 2 Diabetes Mellitus (T2DM), but there are other forms including gestational diabetes, maturity onset diabetes of the young (MODY) and others.

One form dominates, however, and that is T2DM. While exact percentages vary slightly from country to country, typically at least 85-95% of all diabetes cases are T2DM.[3] This is the form associated with obesity and an unhealthy lifestyle. The remaining proportion is primarily those people living with T1DM, while other subtypes are rarer still.

Complications and Costs

Diabetes is a particularly nasty long-term condition because of the complications associated with it. However, these can often be avoided if the disease is managed well, and people living with diabetes can often lead long and healthy lives. If managed poorly though, that's when complications occur. These are often traumatic – diabetes is the most common cause of leg amputations across the world, for instance, with more than 1 million people losing a leg every year.[4] That's one lost leg every thirty seconds.

The psychological impact of limb loss is immense, but this is just one of many possible serious complications. Others include an increased risk of vision loss (diabetic retinopathy), kidney disease (diabetic nephropathy), cardiovascular disease, and degenerative brain diseases such as Alzheimer's disease. In the UK around 1 in 4 patients living with T2DM suffer from coronary heart disease, and around 1 in 10 suffer from stroke.[5] An additional complication, which isn't talked about as often, is the more delicate issue for men living with diabetes; approximately 32% of T1DM male patients and 46% of T2DM male patients suffer from erectile dysfunction.[6]

Living with diabetes comes at a heavy physical and mental cost for the individual, but diabetes also comes with a heavy economic cost for global societies. This is due both to direct treatment costs, as well as indirect costs such as loss of work and wages. The Imperial College London study calculated that the direct cost of diabetes across the globe in 2014 was an eye-watering $825 billion.[7] The biggest contributors to this number were China ($170 billion), the USA ($105 billion), India ($73 billion), and Japan ($37 billion). These numbers don't even begin to take into account the indirect costs associated with the disease. The majority of the direct economic costs associated with diabetes are not actually down to treating the disease with diabetes-specific medication either, but from the complications, particularly cardiovascular problems.

A study by the London School of Economics set out to quantify the costs of diabetes for the EU5 countries (France, Germany, Italy, Spain, UK). As you can see in the table below, diabetes medication represents a small proportion of the overall cost associated with the disease.

TABLE 1 The cost of diabetes for five European Countries (2012 report)

	Germany	UK	France	Italy	Spain
Total Medication Cost	20%	22%	27%	30%	47%
Diabetes Medication	-	7%	6%	6%	10%
Non-diabetes Medication	-	15%	21%	23%	36%
Inpatient Cost	34%	66%	38%	57%	36%
Outpatient Cost (without medication)	28%	9%	36%	14%	17%
Other	19%	2%	-	-	-
Total Cost Per Year	**€43 Billion**	**€20 Billion**	**€13 Billion**	**€8 Billion**	**€5.5 Billion**
Average Cost Per Patient	**€5.9k**	**€5.5k**	**€5.4k**	**€2.8k**	**€1.7k**

The majority of the costs are due to inpatient and outpatient hospital visits due to complications associated with the disease. Some of the most costly complications include:

Haemodialysis:	€41k (Spain) – €81.5k (France) per year[8]
Renal transplant:	€33k (UK) – €77k (Germany)[9]
Amputation:	€17k (UK)[10]

The list of possible complications is so long, however, that it is difficult to estimate the exact cost of diabetes as a whole. It is often not possible even to unpick the precise number of complications that are attributed to diabetes and those that are unrelated. A number of different methods can be used to estimate total cost, and these estimates can also vary significantly from scientific study to study as a result. The magnitude of the cost also differs considerably between and within countries, as does the amount of data available to make these calculations.

Nevertheless, given the general under-reporting of diabetes-related complications and costs by countries, it's likely that the true financial impact of diabetes is even higher than we imagine.

Prevalence Over Time

The prevalence of diabetes has increased enormously since the 1980s. The following tables provide a breakdown of how numbers have grown over the last 35 years for different countries. As you can see, this is not a disease exclusive to western developed nations, but a truly global problem.[11, 12]

TABLE 2 The increased incidence of diabetes by continent between 1980 and 2014.

	Prevalence (%)		Number (millions)	
	1980	2014	1980	2014
African Region	3.1%	7.1%	4	25
Region of the Americas	5.0%	8.3%	18	62
Eastern Mediterranean	5.9%	13.7%	6	43
European Region	5.3%	7.3%	33	64
South-East Asia Region	4.1%	8.6%	17	96
Western Pacific Region	4.4%	8.4%	29	131

The authors of this study went one step further by evaluating the age-adjusted increase in diabetes prevalence. This is an important calculation because T2DM is strongly associated with age, so you would naturally expect the number of people with diabetes to increase with an aging population. Age-adjusted calculations take this in account, and show the net change in diabetes prevalence. The authors calculated that global age-standardised diabetes prevalence between 1980 and 2014 increased from 4·3% to 9·0% in men, and from 5·0% to 7·9% in women, which leads us to infer that a number of factors about our modern lifestyles are responsible beyond age alone. Diet, exercise, sleep, and stress management all play their role. If current trends continue, over 700 million adults across the planet will be living with diabetes by 2025.[13]

The importance of prevention

The challenge is to stem the overwhelming tide of people developing T2DM. Prevention is at once entirely possible and absolutely critical, but when you look at the number of people at high risk of T2DM, the enormity of the task can seem almost overwhelming.

One of the most common methods of identifying people at risk in the western world is with a blood test that analyses the amount of glycated HbA1c in a person's blood. Over time, glucose irreversibly binds to proteins in HbA1c through a process called glycation. Given that your blood cells live for around 120 days, the glycated HbA1c test essentially gives you an average of your blood sugar levels over the last 3 months. High HbA1c readings indicate high levels of blood sugar over a sustained period of time, a hallmark of T2DM.

The US defines people at risk of T2DM if their glycated HbA1c is over 5.7%, while the WHO defines it as over 6.0%. The 0.3% difference between thresholds produces wildly different estimates of the numbers of people at risk.

Using the US definition, it is estimated that almost 1 in 3 people are at risk of T2DM in the US[2] and UK[14], whereas the slightly more lenient WHO definition reduces that number to around 1 in 12 people in the UK.[15] Regardless of which definition you choose to use however, the number of people at risk is huge.

There are other methods to identify people at risk of T2DM aside from the HbA1c test. One method commonly favoured worldwide, partly due to a lack of available HbA1c data, is the Impaired Glucose Tolerance test. A patient is diagnosed with Impaired Glucose Tolerance when:

1. Their blood glucose levels are relatively normal after fasting e.g. first thing in the morning;

2. When the patient is given 75 g of glucose (e.g. a sports drink), their body clears the glucose out of their blood relatively slowly.

The second criteria indicates a level of insulin resistance, which is one of the main factors associated with T2DM.

Using the impaired Glucose Tolerance definition, the International Diabetes Federation (IDF) estimated that 318 million people worldwide were at high risk of developing T2DM in 2015.[16] They reported that North America and the Caribbean had the highest prevalence (13.9% age adjusted), while Europe had the lowest (4.1% age-adjusted). The following table shows the top 10 countries by number of people at risk of T2DM, according to the IDF:

TABLE 3 The number and proportion of people at risk of T2DM by continent.

Rank	Region	% at risk of T2DM (age-adjusted)	Number (millions)
1	North America & Caribbean	13.9%	52
2	Africa	9.1%	35
3	Middle East & North Africa	8.6%	30
4	South & Central America	8.0%	42
5	Western Pacific	6.0%	102
6	South-East Asia	4.7%	42
7	Europe	4.1%	32

Despite the huge numbers at risk, the good news is that T2DM is almost entirely preventable. As has already been mentioned, 85-95% of all T2DM cases are directly attributable to an unhealthy lifestyle.[17, 18] The European Medical Journal reiterated this in one of their reviews of diabetes prevention programmes: "landmark diabetes prevention studies show that lifestyle intervention, focusing on increases in physical activity, improvements in diet, and reductions in weight, reduces the risk of progression to T2DM by 30-60%".[19]

What's Needed?

So we know what we need to do. We need to help those already living with diabetes to live a healthier lifestyle in order to reduce their risk of developing the devastating complications associated with the disease. We also need to prevent as many people as possible from getting T2DM in the first place.

This chapter closes with a brief look at the challenges faced with prevention, for which there are two main approaches:

- **Screen and treat approach**: provide intensive diabetes prevention programmes to individuals at high risk of the disease;

- **Population-wide approach**: implement new public health policies designed to improve overall population health, and therefore reduce overall diabetes prevalence.

The UK, Australia, and US are primarily focusing on screen and treat approaches. The UK recently launched their National Diabetes Prevention Programme (NDPP), for example. Nevertheless, one of the main challenges with the 'screen and treat' approach is successfully identifying those people at risk.

A publication in the British Medical Journal in early 2017 concluded that the diagnostic accuracy of a number of different tests used to identify people at risk of T2DM is low.[20] When discussing the glycated HbA1c test in particular, the authors concluded that the test is neither sensitive, nor specific. They argued that the HbA1c test fails to reliably identify those people at high risk of T2DM (sensitivity), while also excluding those at low risk (specificity).

Even though there isn't complete agreement on how best to define and detect those at risk of T2DM, screen-and-treat polices appear to be the best option for the immediate future. While population-wide health policies are certainly needed, they are unlikely to stem the tide of the T2DM epidemic alone, and often take many years to implement and validate.

To prevent diabetes, the individual concerned needs to sustainably change their behaviours and improve their lifestyle. This is often best achieved through the combination of multiple behavioural change techniques – including social support, structured-education, and personalised goal-setting.

Despite the rapid increase in diabetes prevalence between 1980 and the present day, we are also living in a promising time of digital proliferation. Whereas some past and current in-person diabetes prevention programmes have often been difficult to implement efficiently and cost-effectively at scale, digital offers a potential avenue to do this. New healthcare technology enables outcome tracking and engages people in their own quantified self. Smartphones allow people to be in regular contact with health coaches and others like themselves for on-going feedback and support.

Alongside this, it is imperative that we get the educational content correct. This includes appropriate education on activity, sleep, stress management, and psychological techniques (e.g., positive psychology). Perhaps most importantly of all, we need to get the nutrition advice right. While there probably isn't just one definitive diet, there are definitely some pieces of nutritional advice that are particularly helpful in reducing your risk of diabetes. On that note, it's time to hand over to the renowned experts in this book to discuss many aspects of diabetes in further detail.

Mike Gibbs

@ourpath_health
ourpath.co.uk

Chapter Two

What is diabetes?

by Dr Malcolm Kendrick

What is diabetes?

If you are going to discuss any disease, the first thing is to attempt to describe what that disease is. Although, you have to be very careful. The word 'disease' may appear to be a straightforward concept. However, when you try to pin it down, it can become much like mercury, slipping away from your fingertips, and disintegrating into a million pieces as you attempt to grasp it. This is perhaps especially true with diabetes.

In this chapter, I shall try to explain what diabetes is, and what may cause it, in as straightforward a way as I can. I also hope to try and highlight some of the errors that have affected almost everyone in the way that they think about this condition. As H.L. Mencken famously said. 'For every complex problem there is a solution that is simple, easy to understand – and wrong.' In the area of diabetes this is most certainly true.

Type 1 Diabetes Mellitus (T1DM)

Diabetes is a Latin word that, literally, means passing a lot of urine. Mellitus means sweet. So, if you pass a lot of sweet smelling, or tasting urine (don't take that thought too far), this is known as diabetes mellitus. This term is still used, although the word 'mellitus' has almost completely fallen from use. Diabetes mellitus has, for almost everyone, simply become diabetes.

It is a condition that was known to the Romans, the Persians the ancient Indians and the Chinese. In the eighteenth century, it was referred to by the physician Thomas Willis as the pissing evil. Evil, it indeed was. Children, for it was almost always children, who started to pass a lot of sweet smelling urine rapidly lost weight, and then died quite shortly afterwards. There was no cure, no treatment, just death.

Some years later, doctors worked out that children with diabetes mellitus were lacking a substance normally produced in the pancreas. A substance that lowered blood sugar levels. They did not know what it was. There is some evidence that people tried feeding children extract of pancreas, but it had no effect. Primarily because insulin is quickly broken down by the acids in the stomach. This is why insulin still cannot be given orally. It must be injected.

It was not until the nineteen twenties that Banting, Best and Macleod managed to isolate insulin. They gave it to a dog, that had been made diabetic by removing its pancreas, and the dog recovered. At least it recovered for a while, before dying shortly after of the other complications that resulted from completely removing the pancreas.

The rest, as they say is history. Banting, Best and Macleod won the Nobel prize. Researchers learned to purify insulin from the recovered pancreases of slaughtered cattle, and pigs. The next breakthrough was the development of synthetic human insulin, which provided better blood sugar control. Whilst Type 1 diabetes does not have a cure, the most devastating effects can now be controlled by regular insulin injections.

This form of 'diabetes' is reasonably straightforward to explain and understand. It starts when the body, for reasons that are still not clear (possibly triggered by a viral infection), attacks the beta-cells in the pancreas, and destroys them. Beta-cells are where insulin is manufactured, and with no insulin available the blood sugar rises very high.

Once the sugar level reaches a certain point, the kidneys can no longer keep hold of it, so the sugar escapes into urine – taking a lot of water with it in the process. Which is why the first sign of diabetes is often a child drinking a lot, and passing a lot of urine.

However, it is not the weight loss, or the passing of lots of urine that is fatal. It is a different process whereby fat cells start to lose hold of their stores of fat (insulin keeps a lid on fat escaping). Fatty acids then tumble into the bloodstream. They are carried to the liver where the liver automatically converts these fats/fatty acids into ketone bodies. (Our metabolism uses ketone bodies for energy in times of relative, or absolute, starvation).

In the absence of insulin, the liver keeps on producing more and more ketone bodies. Because ketone bodies are acidic, the entire bloodstream becomes increasingly acidic. Once the body's buffering systems have been overwhelmed, children fall into a keto-acidotic coma – then die. Having first lost most of their fat stores and turned into virtual skeletons.

Type 2 Diabetes Mellitus (T2DM)

From very early times it was also known that it was not only very thin children who produced too much sweet smelling urine. There were also adults who produced too much sweet urine. However, they were usually fat instead of thin. They did not immediately die either. So, whilst they also had (by definition) diabetes mellitus, there was clearly something very different going on.

At first, not many people were very interested in 'fat diabetes'. It was 'thin diabetes' that took up most of the attention of early researchers. Indeed, it was not until 1936 that the difference between the two types of diabetes was clearly established by Sir Harold Percival (Harry) Himsworth. He made it clear that there are two distinct types of diabetes. Type 1 and Type 2.

Unfortunately, the naming of these two forms of diabetes was not fixed at that point, and it underwent many changes over the years. There was an attempt to differentiate the two forms of diabetes as: 'juvenile' and 'adult onset diabetes', also 'Type A and Type B' diabetes, insulin dependent and non-insulin dependent diabetes – and a few others. At one point there was LADA (latent onset diabetes of adulthood) that seems to have fallen out of favour. We also have maturity onset diabetes of youth (MODY), which seems somewhat of a contradiction in terms.

The reason for all this chopping and changing is that these naming systems did not work. It was fully possible to find older people developing juvenile type diabetes and, increasingly, juveniles developing adult onset diabetes. In addition, many adult onset diabetics required insulin to keep their blood sugar levels under control. Eventually the world returned to the idea of calling diabetes Type 1 and Type 2. Hopefully, not too many more changes in the future.

With Type 1 and Type 2 diabetes we still have two diseases that could, accurately, be called diabetes mellitus. However, the underlying disease process is completely different. In Type 2 diabetes, at least in the early stages, there is no lack of insulin production. Often there is more insulin produced than in those without diabetes. However, the insulin fails to have the effect on blood sugar levels that would be expected.

Many people have stated that this means there must be insulin resistance. In fact, Type 2 diabetes is often called 'insulin resistant' diabetes. Whilst this must be, to an extent, true, it does not help much, if at all, in trying to explain what is actually happening. As I will attempt to explain later on.

The health and economic problems with Type 2 diabetes mellitus (T2DM)

For a long time, doctors were not that concerned about T2DM as a sinister health condition. Very few people were monitored for their blood sugar levels, and there was not much in the way of treatment. This all began to change when it was noted that those with T2DM had a greatly increased risk of heart attacks and strokes, otherwise known as cardiovascular disease (CVD). This was true of both men and women; indeed diabetes seems to wipe out female protection against CVD.

In relatively quick succession, a number of other studies confirmed the CVD link, and added in whole series of other health problems. Such as retinal damage and potential blindness, also an increase risk of kidney failure, peripheral artery disease, peripheral neuropathy (damage to nerves) and suchlike. The list is long.

It became clear that, whilst T2DM (which I shall now call diabetes) was not as rapidly fatal as T1DM, it was clearly a serious medical condition, one that was crying out for treatment. It has also become far more common. Indeed, we are in the midst of what has been called a diabetes epidemic.

Early figures on the prevalence of diabetes are unreliable – mainly because people were not being screened. However, it is beyond doubt that it is becoming increasingly common. It is currently estimated to affect around six per cent of the population in the UK, which is a total population of around six million. The cost of treating diabetes has been put at ten per cent of the total NHS budget. Which is around fourteen billion pounds each year.

In the US, the total cost of treatment has been put at two hundred and forty-five billion dollars every year. Equivalent to the entire gross domestic product of Israel. Many people fear that the medical management of diabetes could bankrupt every single healthcare system in the future.

How does it develop

Diabetes develops relatively slowly. You do not wake up one morning to find that you have got diabetes. For example, it has been known for many years now that women who are pregnant can develop 'gestational diabetes.' That is, a high blood sugar level that reveals itself during pregnancy, then goes away again after the birth.

Gestational diabetes normally returns in any subsequent pregnancy, and goes away again. Then, some years later, the woman will probably be diagnosed with diabetes. It appears from this, that pregnancy reveals an underlying progressive problem.

This slow(ish) progression is true of almost everyone else, and it usually goes through different stages. The first stage, before there are any symptoms, or any other signs, is an increased insulin response to a glucose test. A glucose test is where you feed someone a defined amount of glucose, usually seventy-five grams. This causes the blood glucose to rise quite rapidly. The sugar level peaks, then falls back to normal within about two hours. That would be considered normal.

If the insulin level rises higher after a standard oral glucose tolerance test (OGTT) this is usually the first sign that diabetes may be on the way. This can probably best be considered to represent the body trying, and succeeding, in overcoming resistance to the effects of insulin*. During this stage the blood sugar levels are normal completely.

- Stage two: The insulin level rises higher, and the blood sugar level rises moderately higher as well. This is often called an impaired OGTT, or simply IGT (impaired glucose tolerance). The blood sugar will fall back to 'normal' though it may take longer to do so than in a perfectly healthy person. The fasting blood sugar will also be normal.

---

* Insulin levels are hardly ever measured in anyone. So, although stage one exists, it is only really a research finding. The average man, or woman, on the street will never know what their insulin level is, and will never know that they are at stage one.

- Stage three: The fasting sugar level is higher than normal. Defined as an impaired fasting glucose level (IFG). The level will not be high enough to be called diabetes. In those with IFG insulin and sugar levels both rise much higher after an OGTT, and take longer to come back down again.

- Stage four: The fasting blood sugar level is high enough to be called diabetes. The OGTT causes a much higher 'spike' in the blood sugar level, and type II diabetes is diagnosed. (At this point the insulin response to the OGTT may become 'burnt out', so the release of insulin will often be lower than expected).

The length of time it takes to travel from 'normal' through stage one to stage four can be decades. It can be much less. We are now seeing more and more children with stage four (frank diabetes), so it can obviously develop quite rapidly.

Of course, these stages are somewhat arbitrary, and the definitions of impaired glucose tolerance moving to impaired fasting glucose are not fixed. The decision as to when you diagnose diabetes also depends on specific glucose levels – which have little basis in any solid data. In fact, as I write, I can guarantee that people will be deciding that the levels of blood sugar used to define diabetes are too high, and should be lowered. The sounds of money tinkles gently in background.

There has already been the relatively recent movement to create the condition known as pre-diabetes. This means that you are not diabetic yet (using the current figures for diagnosis), but you soon will be. This process is primarily driven by pharmaceutical companies who are desperate to 'treat' ever lower blood sugar levels with life-long medication.

Of course, to an extent, the pharmaceutical companies are right. Why do we only try to treat people at the point when their blood sugar reaches some arbitrary point? Surely we should be treating them earlier to stop them reaching this point in the first place. Well that makes sense…. But only if it works.

Equally, most people with some level of impaired glucose tolerance usually have other, potentially damaging things, going on. This was first really highlighted by Gerald Reaven. He recognised that a number of people who had raised blood sugar levels, but who were not yet diagnosed with diabetes, had a consistent spectrum of metabolic and physiological abnormalities. Sometimes called the metabolic syndrome: To quote Wikipedia:

'The main sign of metabolic syndrome is central obesity (also known as visceral, male-pattern or apple-shaped adiposity), overweight with adipose tissue accumulation particularly around the waist and trunk.

Other signs of metabolic syndrome include high blood pressure, decreased fasting serum HDL cholesterol, elevated fasting serum triglyceride level (VLDL triglyceride), impaired fasting glucose, insulin resistance, or prediabetes.

Associated conditions include hyperuricemia, fatty liver (especially in concurrent obesity) progressing to nonalcoholic fatty liver disease, polycystic ovarian syndrome (in women), erectile dysfunction (in men), and acanthosis nigricans (dark lines on the skin).'

In fact, there are a whole series of other abnormalities as well. Such as increased blood clotting factors, high levels of inflammatory markers, high levels of ceremides and diglycerols... the list is long.

Just to confuse the picture a little more, metabolic syndrome has gone by a number of other different names:

- Reaven's syndrome

- Syndrome X

- Pre-diabetes

- Insulin resistance syndrome

Whatever it was, or is, called, it is clear that there are stages before frank Type 2 diabetes is diagnosed, where serious damage is already being done. Various researchers have found that those with the metabolic syndrome have nearly the same risk of CVD as people with diabetes.

Here is a short quote from a paper called *'Metabolic syndrome and risk of cardiovascular disease: a meta-analysis.'*

'This analysis strongly suggests that the metabolic syndrome is an important risk factor for cardiovascular disease incidence and mortality, as well as all-cause

mortality. The detection, prevention, and treatment of the underlying risk factors of the metabolic syndrome should become an important approach for the reduction of the cardiovascular disease burden in the general population.[1]

Perhaps we should rename diabetes completely. Instead of IGT (impaired glucose tolerance) IFG (impaired fasting glucose) and then diabetes. We should call this metabolic condition stage 1, 2 or 3 diabetes. Maybe I should not suggest this, as the pharmaceutical companies will soon be out with even more medications, to be used even earlier. Then we will all be bankrupt.

In fact, at one time there *was* an attempt to define metabolic syndrome as a disease. I am not quite sure how one creates a disease from a syndrome. I think you just keep saying it often enough until it happens. I presume that the plan was to find a treatment for metabolic syndrome. To quote:

Most people may not have heard of metabolic syndrome, but that is likely to change. Once known mysteriously as syndrome X, the condition, a precursor to heart disease and type 2 diabetes, is about to be transformed into a household name by the US pharmaceutical industry and its partners in the medical profession. A society dedicated to addressing the condition has been organised, a journal has been started, and an education campaign launched. Patients are already being tested for metabolic syndrome. As the trade publication Pharmaceutical Executive said in its January 2004 issue: 'A new disease is being born.'[2]

Since then… nothing much has been heard of this initiative. Why not? Well, if the metabolic syndrome is the underlying problem in a whole series of other conditions, and it probably is, then if the metabolic syndrome went away, all of the associated conditions would simply go away too. No more high blood pressure, low HDL and high VLDL (dyslipidaemia), obesity, impaired blood glucose levels fatty liver, erectile dysfunction etc. etc.

Thus, if you actually managed to cure metabolic syndrome, about half the medications prescribed around the globe would no longer be needed. Tens of millions of people would no longer need high blood pressure medication. The market for T2DM would shrivel up and die. Pharmaceutical company profits would be annihilated overnight. So, we hear little about metabolic syndrome anymore.

However, despite the rapid rise and subsequent disappearance of the metabolic syndrome, it does raise a critical issue. Namely that diabetes is far from a simple condition where the blood sugar level is high – end of. A whole range of other potentially damaging factors are deranged at the same time. Any, or all of which could cause the health problems associated with diabetes. Perhaps the blood sugar level doesn't really matter at all. It is just a marker for underlying metabolic dysfunction.

I am not saying that this is necessarily the case, but the possibility does not even seem to be considered. At present the very strong impression given, and unconsciously accepted, is that diabetes is almost entirely about blood sugar levels, and insulin. If the sugar is high, this is bad. If it is low, this is good. On the other hand, insulin is good, because it lowers blood sugar levels.

This simple meme was evolved to a large extent after the discovery of the role of insulin in Type 1 diabetes. Children who have diabetes have a lack of insulin. If you give them insulin, their sugar levels fall, and they become well again. Thus it has been accepted that sugar is bad, insulin is good. However, it was never the high sugar levels that killed them. It was the keto-acidosis caused by fatty acids escaping from adipose tissue. A completely different metabolic problem. And, of course, if your blood sugar level falls too low, this will kill you quicker than anything else. Sugar bad?

The treatments for T2DM

As you might expect almost all of the treatments for diabetes focus on increasing insulin levels, or trying to overcome the build-up of resistance to the effects of insulin in two organs, the liver and skeletal muscle (what you or I would call muscle). For these are the only two parts of the body where a problem, if it can be called a problem, exists.

Muscles can store glucose, about one thousand calories in an average sized person. Glucose is stored as glycogen (lots of glucose molecules stuck together as a 'polymer'). This reduces the amount of water needed to surround each glucose molecule. The liver can store about five hundred calories, also as glycogen.

So, three mars bars and your sugar/glycogen stores are full. Once this happens the liver switches on a different system, known as lipogenesis (the creation of fat). Thus, after a high carbohydrate

45

meal, if your glycogen stores are full, the liver will start producing fat, from glucose. It will then send this excess fat out, wrapped up in triglycerides (also known as very low density lipoproteins VLDL) – as these lose fat, they shrink down to become LDL (low density lipoproteins a.k.a. 'bad' cholesterol).

Moving back to the main theme here. Resistance to the effects of insulin in muscle and the liver starts when both organs have sufficient glucose/glycogen stores and cannot store any more. You could say that this is not resistance, per-se, it is just the liver and muscle being full and redirecting energy storage to fat instead of sugar. To be stored in adipose tissue (fat cells).

Anyway, with regard to the drugs used to treat diabetes, we have metformin – the most commonly used. This helps to reduce release/ formation of glucose, from glycogen, from the liver (gluconeogenesis), and increases insulin sensitivity in the muscles. We also have sulphonylureas, there are many of these, which flog the beta-cells to produce more insulin. We have pioglitazone, which is supposed to increase insulin sensitivity in muscle and does something beneficial in the liver.

We have acarbose, which stops the body digesting carbohydrates (which are all turned to sugar in the gut). We have other new drugs that increase hormones produced in the gut which stimulate insulin production after eating – in various ways. The most recent drugs are those that prevent the kidneys from reabsorbing sugar, so more sugar is lost in the urine. Hmmmm.

As you can see these are all focussed on insulin, and sugar, and nothing much else. Finally, of course, we have insulin itself. More and more people with T2DM are put on insulin to keep the blood sugar down. Of course, people are also told to lose weight and exercise more. People have been told to do this for the last forty years. Obesity and diabetes have both exploded in the past forty years. So this advice has been splendidly effective.

Another form of treatment, or management, for diabetes is the advice to eat a low fat, high carbohydrate diet. On the surface this may seem mad. Whilst carbohydrates come in many different forms, from wood, to lobster shells, to grains and potatoes and rice and pasta and suchlike, they are all made of simple sugars, e.g. glucose and fructose.

When these simple sugars are bound together, in complex forms, they can become solid, and difficult to break down. So humans cannot eat wood, for example, because we cannot break down the bonds between the sugars. Woodworm, however, can eat wood. Cows can eat grass – we cannot – as our digestive systems can do nothing with grass. Indeed, apart from simple sugars we struggle to break down any complex carbohydrates. Try eating an uncooked potato and see what happens.

Of course, if you cook carbohydrates e.g. beans, or pasta, or potatoes, or most vegetables, this heating breaks down the bonds between the sugars and allows us to eat, and digest them. The process of digesting means breaking them down into glucose and fructose which then enters our bloodstream, where these simple sugars travel to the liver. Where the liver will do various things to them.

Thus, if we eat carbohydrates, we are effectively eating sugar. As a high blood sugar level is considered the problem in diabetes – why would we advise people with diabetes to eat sugar? This seems counter-intuitive.

The answer is that two thoughts combined some years ago. First, it was 'known' that a high fat/saturated fat diet increases cholesterol levels and increases the risk of cardiovascular disease. (I do not believe this). Then it was found that people with diabetes have a greatly increased risk of cardiovascular disease. Ergo, people with diabetes should avoid eating fat at all costs. So people with diabetes eat a high carbohydrate diet.

Indeed, NHS advises people with diabetes, to base meals around food with starchy carbohydrate such as:

- Potatoes

- Cereals

- Pasta

- Rice

- Bread

Well and truly bonkers.[3]

What causes diabetes?

Here is where the territory becomes more difficult. Before starting I feel I must begin with one of my favourite quotes on the possible causes for diabetes. It comes, once again, from the NHS.

'Your risk of developing type 2 diabetes is also increased if your blood glucose level is higher than normal, but not yet high enough to be diagnosed with diabetes.'[4]

Really! How amazing. If you have a high blood sugar level, you are more likely to end up with an even higher blood sugar level – than someone with a normal blood sugar level. Another gem comes from diabetes.co.uk

'Another theory put forward by scientists into how obesity could lead to type 2 diabetes is that obesity causes prediabetes, a metabolic condition that almost always develops into type 2 diabetes.'[5]

Ho hum… we are surrounded by flipping geniuses.

Cutting through circular logic, the current thinking is that obesity is the main cause of diabetes. This is what almost everyone thinks. Most doctors have a model in their brains that looks something like this:

You eat too much/exercise too little → obese → insulin resistance → diabetes

This is another reason why everyone, including people with diabetes are told to avoid fat. Fat contains nine calories of energy, per gram (9 kcal/g). Sugar/carbohydrates, contain around four calories per gram (4 kcal/g). So, if you eat a hundred grams of fat, you will have eaten nine hundred calories of energy. One hundred grams of carbohydrate gives you four hundred calories etc. So you can eat more carbs and put on less weight (or maybe not), and as weight = diabetes risk, carbs must be the way to go (or maybe not).

However, I would like to take you on a detour, or a different way of thinking. Starting with an article in the New York Times entitled: *'Skinny and 119 pounds, but with the health hallmarks of obesity.'*

'Clare Walker of Queens was a medical mystery. No matter how much she ate, she never gained any weight. And yet Ms Walker, with a long narrow face, had

the conditions many obese people develop. Diabetes, raised blood pressure, raised cholesterol, and most strikingly, a liver buried in fat.'[6]

A very thin woman with the most severe insulin resistance her doctor had ever seen. What was going on? What was going on was that she has a condition called lipodystrophy. Very rare indeed. A condition whereby the body has no fat cells (or virtually no fat cells). In this case we have a model that goes as follows:

No fat cells → insulin resistance → diabetes

Try, if you can, to fit those two models together in a way that works. Initially, you would think that one of them must be wrong. It is always tempting to ignore the 'unusual.' Just forget about lipodystrophy, you can learn nothing from that! We know that obesity caused diabetes, so finding completely thin people with diabetes is just the exception that proves the rule.

No, it is not. Those with lipodystrophy actually help to explain diabetes. It is usually at the extremes where the answers can be found.

In lipodystrophy there are no fat cells. Therefore, when people with this condition eat food what happens? Well, clearly there is nowhere for it to go. Fifteen hundred calories stored as glycogen (glycogen stores are now full). Some protein going into muscles (protein stores full). Fat going…. Going where? Well, nowhere – apart from the liver.

Essentially, people with lipodystrophy are very rapidly full up. A problem further compounded by the fact that, without fat cells there is no leptin produced. Leptin is a powerful signal released by fat cells, that travel to the brain to tell us to stop eating. With no leptin those with lipodystrophy are hungry all the time.

Imagine Ms Walker eats ten doughnuts. A thousand calories of carbohydrate. The insulin level skyrockets, the liver tries to convert the sugar to fat – but the liver is already full of fat – with nowhere else to go. Now, is this woman insulin resistant, or simply full up? I would say she is simply full up. In fact, she first went to the doctor with lumps on her skin, that turned out to be cholesterol crystals building up. Yes, there was nowhere for cholesterol to go either. (No heart disease though).

Using people such as Ms Walker as a model, researchers have gone on to create mice with lipodystrophy. Guess what, with absolutely no fat cells, they are all diabetic too. But researchers have gone on to do something with the mice that they cannot do to humans. They implanted fat into these 'fat free' mice. At which point the diabetes and all other metabolic abnormalities simply went away.

So it could be said that, in this case, obesity cured their diabetes. Would this happen in humans too? Almost certainly. With more and more fat cells available, sugar is converted to fat, fat is then stored in fat cells. The fatty liver disappears, the high blood sugar levels disappear, and the insulin levels fall back to normal.

So what, you might think, is actually going on with diabetes?

What we have is something that is both complex, and simple. Complex in that many other hormones have a role to play. Glucagon, cortisol, growth hormone etc. I am not going to cover what they do in any detail here. Complex in trying to establish, what is the actual process by which organs (the liver and muscle) end up resistant to the effect of insulin. Molecules such as diglycerides and ceramides have an effect on glucose transport. Again, I am not going there in one short chapter.

But also simple, in some ways. Simple if you think of insulin as the energy storage hormone. Yes, it lowers blood sugar levels. But this is not the primary function. It is perfectly possible to remove all the beta-cells from the pancreas – without seeing any effect on blood glucose levels. If, that is, you also remove all the alpha-cells. Cells where glucagon is produced. Glucagon is the sugar level raising hormone.

If we look at insulin as the energy storage hormone, we can re-think diabetes in a simple fashion. When we eat more calories than we need, insulin organises the body to store it away in the most efficient way possible. Which, basically means storing it in fat cells. So long as there are enough fat cells in the body, energy can be stored, almost forever. No fatty liver, no increased blood sugar levels, none of the other damaging molecules seen in the metabolic syndrome.

However, once the body is full, once it is struggling to make more fat cells, we get back pressure. This back pressure is exactly the same as we see in people like Ms Walker. When there is nowhere left for energy to be stored, and all hell breaks loose.

We see this in PIMA Indians. The population with the highest rate of diabetes in the world. (They live in North Mexico and Southern US states). In this population there is a high level of insulin produced very early on to a standard glucose tolerance test. These people become obese very rapidly, then they become diabetic. But the first problem is excess insulin production. So with the PIMA, the model is:

Increased insulin production → obesity → insulin resistance → diabetes

Here, it is increased insulin that is the problem. Too much insulin production means that energy is stored as fat very quickly and efficiently. This leads to obesity, then insulin resistance, then diabetes. In short, insulin is not the solution to diabetes, it is the problem. Too much insulin makes people obese.

And what substance raises insulin levels more than any other? The answer is carbohydrates. Thus, if you eat a high carbohydrate diet, you will store fat quickly and efficiently. You will become obese, insulin resistant and, eventually diabetic. If you are already diabetic and you eat a high carbohydrate diet, you will become more obese, more insulin resistant. and more severely diabetic.

It is all, in one way, very simple indeed.

Dr Malcolm Kendrick

@malcolmken
drmalcolmkendrick.org
The Great Cholesterol Con, John Blake Publishing Ltd, 2007
Doctoring Data: How to sort out medical advice from medical nonsense, Columbus Publishing Ltd, 2014

Chapter Three

What causes Type 2 diabetes?

by Dr Jason Fung

High blood glucose is the most obvious clinical feature of the Type 2 Diabetes Mellitus (T2DM), but it is only a symptom of disease and not the disease itself. So, what *is* T2DM? What causes it? What is the etiology of T2DM?

This is a crucial question. Without understanding the cause, it is impossible to devise a rational treatment. T2DM is accepted as a disease of excessive insulin resistance, which causes the high blood glucose readings that characterise the disease. This immediately suggests an important conundrum. If the problem is high insulin resistance, then why is treatment entirely directed towards correcting the high blood glucose?

It is far more logical and effective to treat the insulin resistance. To do so, we must understand what causes this insulin resistance.

Insulin Resistance

Insulin is a normal hormone produced when we eat and it allows glucose to move from the blood into the cells. The cell wall normally prevents glucose from moving freely into the cell from the blood. Glucose enters through specialised gates that may open and close depending upon the level of insulin.

Insulin attaches to the cell by binding to surface receptors, much like a lock and key. Insulin (the key) fits snugly into the corresponding receptor (lock), which opens the door allowing glucose to enter easily.

Insulin also directs the flow of energy. When we eat, there is more energy immediately available than we can use. Insulin directs some of the energy to be used directly by the cells, and the surplus is put into storage – either as glycogen in the liver, or as fat.

When we stop eating, insulin levels fall. The low insulin levels signals the liver to start releasing some of this stored food energy.

In T1DM, destruction of the pancreatic insulin producing cells results in constant, very low insulin levels. Without insulin, the body continually breaks down stores of food energy (glycogen and fat) and turns it into glucose. This glucose piles up outside the cell in the blood, causing the classic symptoms of excessive thirst and urination.

T2DM is entirely different. Insulin levels are not low, but instead are very high levels. There is plenty of insulin around, but it is not working very well. This is called 'insulin resistance' and results in glucose piling up in the blood. To compensate, the body produces more insulin. The insulin is still not working properly, but the higher amount of hormone allows the resistance to be 'overcome' and glucose is forced to enter the cell.

But what caused the insulin resistance in the first place?

Is the problem the insulin, or the insulin receptor? Well, neither. In Type 2 diabetics, the structure of insulin and the insulin receptor are completely normal. Classically, we imagine that something interferes with the gate mechanism, much as some gum in the lock might do. This gummed up lock prevents the key from opening the gate. Less glucose enters the cells causing a state of 'internal starvation'. The body's knee-jerk reaction is to increase production of insulin.

But what is gumming the system? All kinds of theories exist. Inflammation. Oxidative Stress. Free radicals. Nobody seems to actually know. This lock and key model sheds no light upon what is causing the insulin resistance. While these may sound impressive, they merely reflect our lack of knowledge. These are total cop-out answers. Inflammation is the body's non-specific response to injury. *But what causes the injury in the first place?* That's the real problem. The inflammation is only the body's response to whatever is causing the injury.

Think about an analogous situation. Suppose we are battlefield surgeons. After decades on the job, we conclude that blood is the major health problem. Every time we see blood, bad things are happening. When we don't see blood, bad things are not happening. It must be the blood that is dangerous. So, deciding that blood is what is killing people, we use leeches to drain people's blood. Genius! The problem, of course, is *what's causing the bleeding*, rather than the blood itself. Look for the root cause. Bleeding is only a marker of disease.

Something (gunshots, knife wounds) causes bleeding, the body's non-specific response to injury. Gunshots cause bleeding, knife wounds cause bleeding, and shrapnel causes bleeding. Those are root causes. The problem is the gunshot, not the bleeding.

The same logic applies to inflammation, oxidative stress or free radicals. All these are non-specific responses to injury. All are simply the markers of disease. Cardiovascular disease, diabetes, neurodegenerative disorders, obesity and cancers all involve chronic inflammation, oxidative stress and free radical formation. But these factors do not cause the disease; they only indicate the *presence* of the disease.

For example, if inflammation were actually a root cause of heart disease, then anti-inflammatory medications (prednisone, ibuprofen, NSAIDs) would be effective in reducing heart disease, or obesity, or cancer. But they are not. If oxidative stress were causing cancer, then antioxidant treatments (Vitamin C, E, or N-Acetylcysteine) would reverse the disease. But they are startlingly ineffective.

Tell me what is *causing* the oxidative stress or inflammation, because these are only responses to injury. Saying "Insulin resistance is caused by inflammation" is like saying "gunshot wounds are caused by bleeding".

Without understanding what causes IR, we have no hope of properly treating it. This lock and key model with 'internal starvation' is a nice story but it cannot explain many of the observations of T2DM. In particular, it fails to explain the central paradox of insulin resistance.

The Central Paradox

Insulin normally helps store incoming food energy. Low insulin levels instruct the liver to release stored glucose into the blood for energy. During insulin resistance, the liver continues to pump out glucose resulting in high blood glucose levels.

In the liver, insulin increases the new production of fat from glucose by stimulating the process of De Novo Lipogenesis (DNL). During feeding, the body must cope with more glucose than can be immediately used. Some is stored as glycogen in the liver, but the amount that can be stored this way is limited. Insulin converts the excess carbohydrate via DNL to fatty acids, which are packaged with glycerol to form triglycerides, the storage form of fat. In essence, the liver converts sugar to new fat.

As the liver becomes more and more resistant to insulin, you should expect that DNL should similarly decrease, due to the state of 'internal starvation'. But in T2DM, DNL not only continues but actually increases. So insulin's effect is *not* blunted but accelerated!

How can the liver be selectively resistant to one effect of insulin yet accelerate the effect of the other? This is happening in the very same cell, in response to the very same levels of insulin, with the very same insulin receptor. The liver is both insulin resistant and insulin super-sensitive at the very same time!

How can we explain this apparent paradox? Obviously, the old 'lock and key, internal starvation' model does not fit the known facts. We desperately need a new paradigm of understanding insulin resistance if we are to have any hope of conquering this disease. So let's go back and think about resistance in a biological system. How do we develop resistance in general?

Exposure creates resistance

The human body is governed by a fundamental biological principle called homeostasis. Our body exists within a certain comfort zone, and will resist change outside of it. For instance, if we become very cold, the body adapts by increasing body-heat generation. If we become very hot, the body sweats to try to cool itself. Adaptability is a prerequisite for survival and generally holds true for all biological systems.

Put a different way, the body develops resistance against whatever is trying to change things. Exposure creates resistance. The body resists cold by generating heat. However, the stimulus for resistance is the cold temperature itself. Let's look at some examples.

Antibiotic resistance

When new antibiotics are introduced, they are extremely effective, but this honeymoon period does not last long. With time and steady use, the antibiotic loses effectiveness, as some bacteria become drug-resistant "superbugs". This situation is not limited to only a few antibiotics, but is a universal problem because it reflects the universal principle of homeostasis.

Exposure creates resistance. Increased antibiotic use naturally selects resistant organisms, which eventually dominate, rendering the antibiotic useless. Our knee-jerk reaction as doctors is to prescribe even more antibiotics to "overcome" the resistance – which backfires, since it only leads to more resistance. Overcoming resistance requires using *fewer* antibiotics, not more. *Persistent, high-level antibiotic use causes antibiotic resistance.*

Viral resistance

Before the development of vaccines, it was common to hold a 'pox party' or sometimes called a 'measles party'. Children with measles or chicken pox would deliberately expose other non-infected children. Fun. Once the children recovered, they would be protected from future infection. Exposure creates resistance.

Vaccines work on exactly the same principle. Edward Jenner understood that milkmaids developed resistance to the fatal smallpox virus because they had contracted the milder but similar cowpox virus. In 1796, he deliberately infected a young boy with cowpox and observed that he was subsequently protected from smallpox. Exposure creates resistance. In this case, *viruses cause viral resistance.* This almost universal tendency again reflects the biological principle of homeostasis.

Drug resistance

When cocaine is taken for the first time, there is an intense reaction – the "high." Repeated hits reduce the intensity of this reaction. Users occasionally take larger and larger doses to achieve the same 'high', creating the potential for addiction.

This same phenomenon is seen in reaction to many therapeutic drugs including narcotics, marijuana, nicotine, caffeine, alcohol, benzodiazepines and nitroglycerin. Exposure creates resistance. In this case, *drugs cause drug resistance.* The solution is not to use more drugs but, almost counterintuitively, to use fewer drugs.

Vicious cycles

The automatic response to the development of resistance is to increase the dosage. For example, in the case of antibiotic resistance, we reflexively respond by using more antibiotics. In the case of drug tolerance, we reflexively use more drugs. In the case of alcohol tolerance, we reflexively use more alcohol. This temporarily "overcomes" the resistance.

But this is also clearly self-defeating. Exposure creates resistance; increased exposure creates only increased resistance. This generates a self-reinforcing cycle – or a vicious cycle. Using higher doses has a paradoxical effect. Using more antibiotics makes antibiotics less effective. Using more cocaine makes cocaine less effective. Using more alcohol makes alcohol less effective. This cycle continues around and around, steadily worsening.

Antibiotics cause antibiotic resistance.

Viruses cause viral resistance.

Drugs cause drug resistance (tolerance).

Exposure creates resistance, but it's not enough. It also needs persistence of those high levels.

Persistence creates resistance

High hormonal levels *by themselves* cannot cause resistance. The pulsatile secretion of hormones prevents the development of resistance. All hormones – cortisol, insulin, growth hormone, parathyroid hormone or any other hormone – are released in bursts. Hormones are released at specific times to produce a specific effect. Afterwards, the levels quickly drop and stay very low.

The body acclimatises quickly when exposed to a constant stimulus. Have you ever watched a baby sleep in a crowded, noisy airport? It is very loud, but constant. The baby is 'resistant' to the noise. Now imagine the same baby sleeping in a quiet house. A slight creak of the floorboards may be enough to wake him up. Even though it is not loud, it is very noticeable.

Hormones work in exactly the same way. Most of the time, hormone levels are low. There is an occasional burst of hormone, which creates maximum effect. After it passes, levels drop to their usual low baseline.

By cycling between low and high levels, the body never gets a chance to adapt. Resistance never develops despite high levels because these levels never persist.

Resistance requires both *high* and *persistent* levels.

Insulin causes insulin resistance

So let's go back to the question we're really interested in. What causes insulin resistance? The first place to search is *persistently high levels of insulin itself.* Many lines of evidence support this argument.

An insulinoma is a rare tumor,[1, 2] which continually secretes abnormally large amounts of insulin in the absence of any other significant disease. As the patient's insulin levels increase, his or her levels of insulin resistance increase in lock step – a protective mechanism and a very good thing. If insulin resistance did not develop, the high insulin levels would rapidly lead to very, very low blood sugars. The resulting severe hypoglycemia would quickly lead to seizures and death. The body protects itself by developing insulin resistance – demonstrating homeostasis. The resistance develops naturally to shield against the unusually large insulin levels. *Insulin causes insulin resistance.*

Surgical removal of the insulinoma dramatically lowers the patient's insulin levels. With the tumor gone, insulin resistance is also dramatically reversed, as well as associated conditions such as acanthosis nigricans.[3] Reversing the high insulin levels (the causal factor) also reverses insulin resistance.

Experimentally, the constant infusion of insulin into a group of normal, healthy, non-diabetic volunteers can easily induce insulin resistance.[4, 5] Within days, insulin sensitivity drops by 20 to 40 percent. The implications are simply staggering. Healthy, young, lean men can be made insulin resistant simply by administering insulin – *which causes insulin resistance.*

High doses of insulin used in T2DM can also induce insulin resistance.[6] In one study patients were started on intensive insulin treatment in order to tightly control blood glucose. In six months, their average insulin dosage increased from zero to 100 units a day.

Blood glucose control was indeed very good. But the more insulin they took, the more insulin resistance they got – a direct causal relationship, as inseparable as a shadow is from a body. Even as the blood glucose was improving, the T2DM was getting worse.

Insulin creates insulin resistance. But insulin resistance also causes high insulin – a classic vicious, or self-reinforcing, cycle. Insulin drives up insulin resistance. This, in turn drives up insulin levels. The cycle keeps going around and around, one element reinforcing the other, until insulin is driven up to extremes.

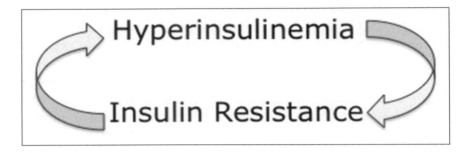

Does high insulin lead to insulin resistance or insulin resistance lead to high insulin levels? The answer is both. One reinforces the other in a vicious cycle. The rich get richer. The fat get fatter. It's an unfair world. The cause of insulin resistance is high persistent levels of insulin itself, also known as hyperinsulinemia.

A new paradigm

How does hyperinsulinemia lead to insulin resistance?

Remember that insulin unlocks the gate that allows glucose to enter the cell. Under conditions of persistently and abnormally high insulin, glucose enters the cell far in excess of energy needs. There's simply too much glucose going into the cell, so it overflows back out into the blood.

From the outside, it appears that the glucose cannot enter the cell and that insulin is not doing its job so this is called 'insulin resistance'. The cell appears resistant to the effect of insulin. It is an *overflow* phenomenon, not a gummed-up lock and key one.

Imagine the cell to be a subway car. Insulin opens the door and the passengers (glucose in the blood) march in a nice orderly manner into the empty subway car (cell). But what happens if there are too many passengers? Insulin opens the door but the passengers cannot enter the subway car and are left at the platform.

If the subway door is gummed up and doesn't open, then the result is the same. But the problem is actually that the subway car (cell) is already overflowing with passengers (glucose). Now the glucose outside the cell simply can't get in and is left crowded on the platform.

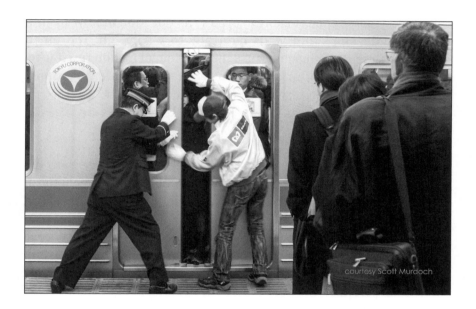
courtesy Scott Murdoch

What can you do?

In Japan, there are attendants who gently push passengers into the trains that are already full. The body's knee jerk reaction is to manufacture more insulin to help push glucose into the cell. Which works, but only for a while.

Like these Japanese subway pushers, insulin tries to push the glucose into the cell. It works, but only to a degree. After a certain point the cell simply cannot accept any more glucose.

The cell is not in a state of 'internal starvation' but is instead overflowing with glucose. One of the most basic principles of toxicology is that the dose makes the poison. Even oxygen in excess is toxic. The same is true for glucose. While some glucose is good, excessive glucose is noxious. Glucose is not toxic, but there's simply too much of it.

The liver feverishly tries to unload itself of the toxic glucose load by converting it into fat via DNL, but this protective mechanism is overwhelmed by the sheer amount of glucose trying to force its way inside. This explains how the cell can appear to be insulin resistant (glucose outside cells) and insulin super-sensitive (enhanced DNL) at the same time. The central paradox of insulin resistance is solved. Mischief managed.

This new paradigm crucially answers the question of how insulin resistance develops and leads naturally to a solution. Too much glucose and too much insulin cause the problem of insulin resistance. Obviously, the ideal solution is to *lower glucose and lower insulin.* Once you lower insulin resistance you can reverse T2DM.

Insulin Resistance is Good?

Everybody assumes that insulin resistance is very, very bad. It's often called the root cause of T2DM and metabolic syndrome. But if it is really so bad, why is it so prevalent? Over 50% of the American population has elevated insulin resistance as manifested by pre-diabetes or diabetes.[7] If it is such a universal reaction, it must serve a protective purpose. Our bodies are not designed to fail. Insulin resistance must serve a protective function, being so common. So how can it be protective?

We accept that excessive glucose in the blood is harmful, but why wouldn't this also be toxic in the tissues of the body, too? Insulin doesn't actually get rid of the glucose but moves it out of the blood and forces it into the tissues.

If you have too much garbage, you need to throw it out, not merely move it around in the same house. The same applies to the excessive glucose. Instead of eliminating the glucose from the body, insulin merely moves it from the blood into the body.

The body will naturally try to protect itself against this excessive glucose load by refusing it. Imagine that you live on a street in DiabetesVille. Each house is like a cell. Insulin normally opens the door to deliver glucose daily. Every day, insulin delivers a little bit of glucose, which the house burns for heat.

Now insulin starts to deliver ten times the normal daily amount. Pretty soon, the houses fill up with glucose. There's just way, way too much. Yet still, everyday insulin comes around to deliver another load of way too much glucose.

After a few years, you'd say, "I don't want all this toxic glucose" and refuse insulin's attempt to deliver more. That's insulin resistance! It's not a bad thing, it's a good thing. Insulin resistance protects the cell from the toxic levels of glucose that the insulin is trying to shove in.

What is Insulin Resistance protecting us *from*? The very name reveals the answer. Insulin Resistance. It's a reaction against *excessive insulin*. The body develops resistance to protect us from the too much insulin. Said another way, insulin causes insulin resistance.

But the primary problem is the excessive insulin, not the insulin resistance. The tissues (heart, nerves, kidney, eyes) are all increasing their resistance to protect themselves from insulin's toxic delivery. The disease is not insulin resistance. The disease is *hyperinsulinemia*.

Back in DiabetesVille, we've refused insulin's attempt to shove glucose into our houses. Glucose is piling up in the streets (the blood). The overflowing glucose is noticed and the body's knee jerk reaction is to increase the insulin, despite that fact that insulin is too high already. This shoves more toxic glucose into the houses (cells), but at least it won't be in the street (blood).

Look! The streets (blood) are nice and clean. But all the toxic glucose has been moved into the cells. We have inadvertently 'overcome' the tissue-protective insulin resistance. Increasing insulin in a situation of excessive insulin only makes things worse.

The toxic agent here is the excessive glucose, and its co-conspirator, insulin. Insulin resistance develops ***precisely*** to protect the cells against the excessive, toxic glucose load. The development of the insulin resistance is universal because it's a *good thing*, not a *bad one*. It's the natural, protective reaction to the root cause – high insulin levels.

It's the insulin, stupid!

The Sugar Bowl

At its very core, T2DM can be understood as too much glucose and too much insulin. The solution becomes immediately obvious. We must lower the insulin and lower the glucose. The sugar is not just in the blood. That's only part of the problem. There's too much sugar in **our entire body**.

63

Imagine our body is a sugar bowl. When we are born, our sugar bowl is empty. Over decades, if we eat too much of the wrong things – sugary cereals, desserts and white bread, the sugar bowl gradually fills until it is completely filled. The next time you eat, sugar comes in, but the bowl is full, so it spills out into the blood.

It's like packing your clothes into a suitcase. At first, the clothes go without any trouble. After a certain point, though, it becomes just impossible to jam in those last 2 T-shirts. You can't close the suitcase. The luggage is now 'resistant' to the clothes. It's much harder to pack those last 2 T-shirts compared to the first two. It's the same overflow phenomenon. The cell is filled to bursting with glucose, so trying to force more in is difficult and requires much higher doses of insulin.

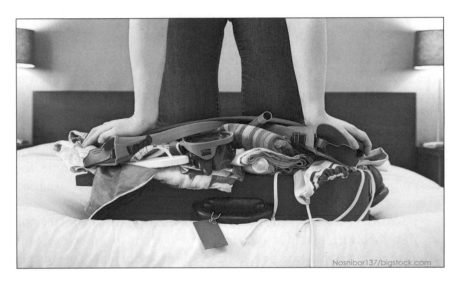

Nosnibor137/bigstock.com

When the insulin levels are unable to keep pace with the increasing resistance, blood sugars rise and T2DM is diagnosed. Your doctor prescribes a medication such as insulin. But insulin does not rid the body of that excess sugar. Instead, it simply takes the blood sugar and rams it back into the liver. The liver doesn't want it either, so it ships it out to all the other organs – the kidneys, the nerves, the eyes, and the heart. Much of this extra sugar will also just get turned into fat.

The problem, of course, has not been solved – the sugar bowl is still overflowing. Insulin has moved sugar from the blood (where you could see it) into the body (where you couldn't see it). The underlying problem is unchanged. So, the very next time you eat, the exact same thing happens. Sugar comes in, spills out into the blood and you inject insulin to cram the sugar back into the body.

This works for a while, but eventually, the body fills up with sugar, too. Now, that dose of insulin cannot force any more sugar into the body. Blood glucose starts to rise again and you go to the doctor.

Instead of getting rid of the toxic sugar load, he doubles the dose of insulin. If your luggage doesn't close, the solution is to empty it out, not use more force. If the cell is overloaded with sugar, you should empty it out, instead of using more insulin to force it in.

The higher dose of medication helps, for a time. Blood sugars go down as you force your body to gag down even more sugar. But eventually, this dose fails as well. Then your doctor gives you ever increasing doses of insulin.

Over a period of years, you move from pre-diabetes, to diabetes taking a single medication, then two then three and then finally large doses of insulin. Here's the thing. If you are taking more and more medications to keep your blood sugars at the same level, your diabetes is getting worse!

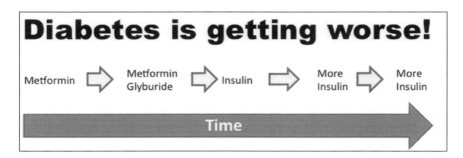

The blood sugars got better with insulin, but the diabetes got worse. This unfortunately happens to virtually every patient. The higher dose of medications only hides the blood sugar by cramming it into the engorged body. The diabetes *looks* better, but actually is getting worse.

Doctors congratulate themselves on the illusion of a job well done, even as patients get continually sicker. Patients require ever-increasing doses of medications and yet still suffer heart attacks, congestive heart failure, strokes, kidney failure, amputations and blindness. "Oh well" the doctor tells himself, "It's a chronic, progressive disease".

Imagine hiding the kitchen garbage under the bed instead throwing it outside in the trash. You can't see it, so you can pretend your house is clean. As the trash piles up, there's no more room underneath the bed, so you throw the garbage into the bathroom, too. You hide it anywhere where you can't see it. Eventually, it begins to smell really, really bad. You need to throw out the garbage, not hide it. That would be a really bad idea.

But we do the exact same thing in the current standard care of T2DM. If we understand that too much sugar in the blood is toxic, why can't we understand that too much sugar in the body is also toxic?

The End Game

What happens over ten or twenty years? Every single part of the body *just starts to rot*.

This is precisely why T2DM, unlike virtually any other disease, affects every single part of the body. Every organ suffers the long-term effects of the excessive sugar load. Your eyes rot – and you go blind. Your kidneys rot – and you need dialysis. You heart rots – and you get heart attacks and heart failure. Your brain rots – and you get Alzheimer's disease. Your liver rots – and you get fatty liver disease and cirrhosis. Your legs rot – and you get diabetic foot ulcers. Your nerves rot – and you get diabetic neuropathy. No part of your body is spared.

Medications and insulin do nothing to slow down the progression of this organ damage, because they do not eliminate the toxic sugar load. We've known this rather inconvenient fact since 2008. No less than 7 multinational, multi-centre, randomised controlled trials of tight blood glucose control with medications (ACCORD, ADVANCE, VADT, ORIGIN, ELIXA, TECOS and SAVOR) have all failed to demonstrate reductions in heart disease, the major killer of diabetic patients. We pretended that using medications to lower blood sugar makes people healthier. But it's only been a lie. All because we've overlooked a singular truth. *You can't use drugs to cure a dietary disease.*

How to Reverse Diabetes

If we understand that T2DM is simply too much sugar, then the solution becomes pretty bloody obvious. Get rid of it. Don't hide it away. Get rid of it. There are really only two ways to get rid of the excessive sugar in the body.

1. Don't put sugar in.

2. Burn it off.

That's it. That's all we need to do. The best part? It's all natural and completely free. No drugs. No surgery. No cost.

Step 1 – Don't put sugar in

The first step is to eliminate all sugar and refined starches from your diet. Sugar has no nutritional value and can be safely eliminated. Starches are simply long chains of sugars. Highly refined starches such as flour or white rice are quickly digested into glucose. The optimum strategy is to eat little or no refined carbohydrates.

Dietary protein is digested into amino acids. Excess amino acids cannot be stored so they are converted into glucose by the liver. Therefore, avoid eating excessive protein as this, too only adds sugar to the body. Protein shakes, protein bars, and protein powders should all be avoided. Instead focus on eating lots of vegetables and natural healthy fats. A moderate intake of protein is optimal.

Dietary fat, long shunned for its purported effect of causing heart disease, is back. Natural fats, such as found in avocado, nuts and olive oil are well known to have healthy effects on both heart disease and diabetes. The Mediterranean diet, high in natural fats is well accepted to be a healthy diet. Dietary cholesterol has also been shown to have no harmful effect on the human body. Eggs and butter are excellent sources of natural fats, which have minimal effect on blood glucose or insulin.

Most importantly, stick to eating whole, natural, unprocessed foods. Low refined carbohydrates, moderate protein and high natural fats.

Step 2 – Burn it off

Fasting is the simplest and surest method to force your body to burn sugar. Blood glucose is the most easily accessible source of energy.

Fasting is merely the flip side of eating – if you are not eating, you are fasting. When you eat, your body stores food energy. When you fast, your body burns food energy. If you simply lengthen out your periods of fasting, you can burn off the stored sugar.

T2DM is merely excessive glucose in the body, so burning it off will reverse the disease. While it may sound severe, fasting has been practiced for at least 2000 years. It is the oldest dietary therapy known. Literally millions of people throughout human history have fasted without problems. If you are taking prescription medications, you should seek the advice of a physician. But the bottom line comes to this.

If you don't eat, will your blood sugars come down? Of course.

If you don't eat, will you lose weight? Of course.

So, what's the problem? None that I can see.

Dr Jason Fung

@drjasonfung
intensivedietarymanagement.com
The Obesity Code: Unlocking the secrets to weight loss, Scribe 2016
The Complete Guide to Fasting, Victory belt 2016

Chapter Four

Who gets Type 2 Diabetes?
(Understanding and treating the causes)

by Dr Robert Cywes

Only two groups of people get Type 2 diabetes (T2DM): drug addicts and performance athletes.

It is neither the addict nor the athlete's fault for becoming diabetic. Remission is possible, but the burdensome responsibility of remission lies solely in the hands of the diabetic and can occur only once they understand why they became diabetic in the first place. I cannot help diabetics to become non-diabetic, but I can help diabetics to help themselves to become so.

Cause of T2DM

T2DM is simply the result of chronic excessive carbohydrate consumption beyond the genetically predetermined maximum carbohydrate handling capacity of the insulin-glucagon hormonal system. Failure of this system to handle excessive carbohydrate consumption causes progressive aberration of the carbohydrate clearance mechanisms resulting in tolerance of increased blood glucose levels above the normally tightly controlled insulin-glucose clamp. T2DM can be put into remission, requiring no medication, with normal diabetic blood indices.

Misconceptions

Obesity does not cause T2DM. T2DM is not a genetic disease and it is not caused by pancreatic dysfunction or a lack of insulin production (T1DM). It is caused by a psychological disorder or misinformation in the case of performance athletes. No medication cures T2DM because medications do not treat the cause of T2DM. Medications only slow down the progression of the disease, merely altering the handling of sugar that is already in the system.

Our Definition of Addiction[1]

Psycho-active endorphin-stimulating substances may be effectively USED in tightly controlled settings to manage a spectrum of daily emotional needs without causing harm. When a person uses pleasure-giving substances in a chronic, excessive and dominant manner, over time the toxic side-effects of the ABUSED substance cause harm. If the person ignores or distorts the reality of that harm to continue the relationship, they lose control of the relationship and have become ADDICTED.

There is no ambiguity that while alcohol is a liquid, its primary role is for psycho-active pleasure not thirst-quenching. There is consensus on the harm of alcoholism and agreement that abstinence is the preferred, if not required, therapy for addicted persons. Alcohol is not a necessity for human survival.

Similar to alcohol or nicotine, carbohydrates are powerful psycho-active, somatotoxic drugs, rather than an essential food source. However, like nicotine addiction in the 1950s and 1960s, society has yet to come to terms with the toxic addictive nature of carbohydrates. The closest we have come is to incorrectly assign the label of "addiction" to food, but real food that has essential nutritive value is non-addictive since it does not activate the endorphin system. It is impossible to develop T2DM or become obese from eating food (i.e. substances that have essential nutritional value). In the spectrum of what we have mislabeled as "food", exclusively carbohydrates are highly addictive[2] and in excess directly or indirectly cause a variety of Chronic Non-Communicable Diseases (CNCDs) including T2DM and obesity. Developing, then ignoring, the cause of these diseases in order to continue the relationship with the drug by definition, is a drug addiction – the drug being carbohydrates.

The psychology of addiction applies equally irrespective of the drug of choice.

As with the treatment of all substance addictions, abstinence (<30 g non-vegetable total carbohydrate consumption per day – see below) from psycho-active use is the preferred, if not required, therapy

70

to induce remission for anyone with a CNCD caused by chronic excessive carbohydrate consumption because by the time a person is obese and/or diabetic, they have lost control of the relationship. Most certainly carbohydrates are not necessary for human survival because blood glucose levels are very effectively maintained by gluconeogenesis and glucagon.

Carbohydrates are an endorphin releasing drug, not a hunger satisfying food.

Human physiology is tightly controlled by numerous genetic feedback pathways. For example, when the thirst centre is activated, and a person drinks water, as soon as thirst is quenched, it shuts down the ability to drink excess water and it is nearly impossible to overdrink water. Water has no action on the endorphin centre. However, if a person is thirsty and starts drinking beer or a sugary drink, the alcohol or sugar powerfully activates the endorphin centre that is not under genetic feedback control, and endorphin activation readily overrides the stopping point of the thirst centre. Therefore, while water consumption is tightly controlled at a subconscious level, alcohol and sugar consumption, although still liquids, has to be consciously controlled. When that control is not exercised, you get drunk or sugar-high and over time, when done repetitively, you lose control of the relationship and you become an alcoholic or a fat diabetic who requires abstinence for effective treatment.

Identically, the hunger centre tightly controls the consumption of essential foods – protein, fat and other essential micronutrients, using neural and hormonal (for example ghrelin and leptin) feedback pathways that are genetically predetermined. No essential nutrient activates the endorphin pathway. Under the control of the hunger-satiety system, it is virtually impossible to overeat essential foods, become unhealthily obese or develop any of the dietary CNCDs such as T2DM that are so prevalent in our society today, since these feedback pathways are designed to protect us as a species.

Carbohydrates, however, are not essential nutrients but powerful endorphin-activating drugs that are not controlled by the genetic hunger-satiety feedback system. At a very early age, the trigger for carbohydrate consumption is hunger or thirst, as part of the genetically-controlled hunger-thirst-satiety feedback system. But when certain people, vulnerable to addiction, are repetitively offered carbohydrates as "food", a stimulus transfer occurs whereby the activator of carbohydrate consumption is no longer mediated by the hydration-nutrition system. Instead, activation transfer occurs to the endorphin system, so that carbohydrate consumption becomes a response to endorphin requirement to manage emotional need rather than a hunger-thirst response to satisfy nutritional need. The requirements of these pathways differ greatly in terms of frequency and quantity, and ultimately repetitive excessive consumption of carbohydrates, beyond the coping capability of the nutritional regulatory system, leads to breakdown of the system resulting in CNCDs that we physicians are now tasked to treat. However, treating the CNCD without addressing carbohydrate consumption, or in fact the psychology of addiction, cannot resolve the disease to the point of remission.

Carbohydrate consumption readily overrides feedback control of both the thirst and the hunger centres and this makes us particularly vulnerable to excessive consumption because of the variety of ways in which the drug can be consumed. Similar to the ubiquitous availability of cigarettes last century, along with denial that smoking caused harm and contributed to the prevalence of smoking-related disease, overconsumption of carbohydrates has been made so much easier by their increased availability in all forms (manufactured, processed and "natural") and the establishment of the misguided belief that they are necessary as part of a healthy diet per the food pyramid of 1977. If humans do not consciously limit their carbohydrate consumption, it is easy to consume them excessively and because carbohydrates in chronic excess disrupt nearly all the essential functional physiological pathways that keep humans healthy, we develop a variety of diseases as these systems become overwhelmed by the toxicity of sugar. In our practice, our data reveals that the average Type 2 diabetic consumes between 75%-90% of all their daily calories as carbohydrates.

Two major errors have further obscured our ability to recognise this causal pathway of T2DM. First, assigning carbohydrates to "more healthy" and "less healthy" categories for diabetics based on the glycemic index concept created by Dr David Jenkins in Toronto and popularised by the McGovern Commission report of 1977.[3] The glycemic index theory made two critical erroneous assumptions: (a) Carbohydrates are essential to human nutrition. Based on this assumption they only compared glycemic index to free unrestricted carbohydrate consumption. They failed to test a third treatment arm – carbohydrate abstinence. (b) humans can reliably control their consumption of carbohydrates, failing to take the concept of addiction into account. Although the glycemic index may experimentally help to stabilise diabetes, following its principles does not put diabetics into remission, and asking someone to tightly control their relationship with a substance they have already lost control of is unfeasible. The Achilles heel of the glycemic index concept can more readily be understood when applied to a similar toxic drug, alcohol. According to glycemic index principles, it would be fine for an alcoholic to drink beer, but not whisky since beer raises your blood alcohol level more slowly, making beer healthy, but whisky not. If abstinence is curative, what value is there in the science of less? Asking a diabetic to count their carbohydrates is no different than asking an alcoholic to count their drinks.

You cannot have T2DM if you do not consume carbohydrates. And just as with alcohol, opioids and nicotine, it matters not how the drug enters your face – whether as a simple sugar or as a complex starch, nor how fast it enters. What matters is how much and how often. Irrespective of the form it takes at entry into your mouth, by the time it enters your bloodstream, it can only be glucose, galactose or fructose.

Secondly, if we as a society are to effectively address T2DM, we first and foremost need to understand the nutritional confusion related to additives. Born of naivety, but now intentionally misleading, it is critical to recognise that additives do not make carbohydrates healthy. A glass of red wine may have healthy anti-oxidant value, but it is not acceptable for an alcoholic to have any because of the concept of permission. Once permission is granted, an alcoholic cannot stop. Similarly, all because we sprinkle a little protein powder on a chocolate bar and call it a "healthbar" or add some electrolytes to a sugar drink and call it Gatorade, or add a few nutrients to fructose and call it an apple, it does not mean it is acceptable for a diabetic to consume it. Many food manufacturers use this clever form of branding to camouflage and sell toxic drugs to us. Starbucks is merely a modern-day Speakeasy, which has done an incredible marketing job of selling sugar occasionally flavoured with coffee. Toxicity occurs at ingestion and, like alcohol for an alcoholic, the first sip or the first chip from the bag is too much and the whole bottle or the whole bag is not enough. T2DM patients need to classify what they consume as healthy or harmful based on the total carbohydrate content not the nutrient additive value. Any substance with a significant total carbohydrate load is toxic to a diabetic irrespective of the glycemic index or the nutritional additives or the label advertisement. Carbohydrates may be a vehicle for consuming essential nutrients, but it is quite easy to access essential nutrients without the carbohydrate load. Essential nutrients can readily be found in real food without the toxic contamination of carbohydrates.

Obesity is associated with, but does not cause T2DM. Both diseases are the consequence of prolonged over-consumption of the same drug – carbohydrates. T2DM manifests as damage to end-organs that result from a series of progressive microvascular injuries due to the toxic effects of chronically elevated blood sugar.[4] Treating the glucose level after the sugar has already entered the bloodstream with exercise or expensive medications may slow down progression of the end-organ damage, but does not affect the disease process. Treating T2DM with medications that whip the pancreas to produce more insulin, or alter blood glucose levels at renal reabsorbtion or provide injectable insulin do not treat T2DM, they merely lower blood glucose. As a society, we are spending billions of dollars on medications that ineffectively clear sugar from the bloodstream when the simplest, most effective way to prevent the disease or put it into remission is by preventing sugar from ever getting into the bloodstream by not putting it into our faces in the first place! So why is this simple preventative action so impossible to achieve? Three reasons: misinformation, addiction and greed.

Misinformation

For endurance athletes that develop insulin resistance and T2DM, the error is simply the scientifically unsupported belief in carbohydrate loading as the primary source of physiologic performance fuel. Perfecting the science of carbohydrate loading is a huge industry, which is so self-sustaining that it dare not ask the first and most fundamental question in medical science: Is carbohydrate loading safe? In our zealousness for enhanced performance, we medical scientists failed to follow our first doctrine – DO NO HARM. The industry itself has become so steadfast in its erroneous belief that carb-loading is essential, that when one of the concept's most ardent developers questioned the foundation of the science, Professor Tim Noakes was maligned to the point of malpractice accusation. However, as Professor Noakes' chapter in this book explains, once athletes alter their diet and change their primary fuel source from carbohydrates to fat consumption – and allow their body systems time to adapt to the new fuel source – their T2DM and related diseases improve remarkably or even go into remission. Such change appears to have a positive impact on performance as well.

Addiction

The overwhelming majority of T2DM is a consequence of carbohydrate addiction. As a society, in order to prevent T2DM and to put the disease into remission, we have to change our focus away from the nutritional value of food and apply the principles of addiction management. At an even more fundamental level, we need to understand and reduce the exponential increase in societal vulnerability to addictive behaviour.

Greed

When you examine the history of any addictive substance, highly pleasurable use begins naively to consequence. Then, as diseases develop due to excessive consumption, societal denial occurs followed by recognition and attempts to address removal of access to the substance. However, by that late stage, so many influential people have made so much money that despite the obvious knowledge of the toxic consequences, the drug remains (freely) accessible in one form or another because greed by a few will always trump the health of the masses. Because of the huge profits to be made in the manufacture, marketing and sale of carbohydrate products, they have become ubiquitously available and relatively inexpensive. However, when you factor into the equation not only the profitability of products sales, but also the broader cost of treating the consequences, the societal economy of carbohydrates results in massive economic loss, not profit. We are repeating a generational species-threatening mistake, smoking and nicotine consumption being the most vivid recent examples. And we still sell cigarettes, don't we.

Who gets T2DM?

Carbohydrates are abundantly and ubiquitously available in our local environment. Why is everyone not fat and diabetic? T2DM requires an intersection between vulnerability to addiction and genetic predisposition to insulin-glucagon dysfunction.

Vulnerability to addiction

The endorphin pathway is a vital human system used to deal with all emotions – stress, boredom, pleasure, anxiety, depression, hypomania. Our understanding is rudimentary and presently characterised by observational behavioural psychology because of our paucity of biochemical and physiologic pathway knowledge.

The human brain can only focus intensely for about 20 minutes at any one time; then it needs a short break to recalibrate. Like windshield wipers on a rainy day, brief frequent activation of the endorphin system provides the mind-cleansing that allows us to refocus. In addition, the human brain requires longer conscious break periods a few times a day where it can rest, relax and process. All humans have a variety of endorphin-activating strategies that are used at various times to relax the brain and deal with emotional needs.

There are two types of endorphin-releasing strategies – action and consumption. The return on the investment of effort is a wonderful sense of relaxation and well-being that provides an endorphin-stimulated arena for contemplation, thought, planning and emotional relaxation and adjustment. For example, physical activity such as going for a walk, human connection sharing a joke or a story, stretching, singing, doodling or painting, praying, meditating. All are powerful endorphin activators that balance the brain but also provide an opportunity to plan ahead and process through emotions in a positive supportive atmosphere. On the other hand, consumption of a psycho-active substance, while powerfully activating the endorphin system, soothes, numbs and obliterates emotions but does not allow for processing, contemplation or planning. Well-adjusted people use a variety of endorphin releasing mechanisms to manage their emotions effectively without harm.

Vulnerability to addiction primarily occurs in two populations – people with authoritarian personalities and people with permissive or hedonistic personalities. While seemingly opposite, both have dysfunctional emotion management systems. The authoritarian group absorb huge amounts of emotional distress from the very mechanism designed to alleviate the emotional distress. They put extra-ordinary effort into all their endeavors, but also set ridiculously high standards. Then, instead of feeling a sense of well–being from the effort, they feel a sense of failure by not meeting the unattainable standard, resulting in an eroded sense of self that finds salvation by triangulation toward an endorphin-releasing substance that in an inanimate manner numbs and soothes but does not process their distress. The permissive group turns away from the option to put effort into their emotional management system where the return of the investment of effort is a sense of well-being and emotional relaxation, and turns toward the more easily attainable substance high, which requires little effort, to deal with their emotional angst. Their self-esteem is low because they diverted away from the effort that in small increments builds a strong sense of self. As these groups selectively use one endorphin-releasing mechanism in a dominant excessive manner, it leads to harm. Occasional consumption of carbohydrates can be a wonderful treat, but when used excessively, as the primary endorphin high, harm happens. Based on genetics, that harm is expressed as one or more of the CNCDs – obesity, hypertension, dyslipidemia, T2DM. Authoritative personality types are not vulnerable to addiction and therefore do not get T2DM.*

Genetic predisposition to T2DM

The pancreas produces insulin in response to carbohydrate consumption. Blood sugar is tightly controlled by the insulin/glucagon response system to maintain blood sugar levels in a tight "clamp" preventing blood sugar from rising too high or falling too low.

---

* This is based on research, led by Diana Baumrind, into parenting styles and impact on personality and behaviors. Baumrind distinguished between authoritarian; permissive and authoritative parenting styles. (Maccoby and Martin added "neglectful" as a style to complement her work.) Authoritarian parents value obedience as a virtue in itself. Authoritative parents are more issue-flexible and pragmatic. The former is a more black and white/right and wrong/all or nothing world; the latter is more grey. As adults, the all or nothing upbringing is more conducive to addiction than the authoritative shades of grey personality.

Simplistically, the maximum amount of insulin the pancreas can produce by stimulation from prolonged or excessive carbohydrate intake is genetically controlled. Some populations (for example East Indians) may have a relatively low upper limit of insulin production, while others have a much larger capacity to produce insulin. We can measure the strain that chronic excessive carbohydrate consumption puts on the pancreas by measuring fasting C-peptide and insulin levels (variably called prediabetes or insulin resistance). Fasting blood glucose and HbA1c levels tell us when a patient is becoming "diabetic" i.e. their insulin-producing capacity can no longer keep pace with carbohydrate consumption and the pancreas loses the ability to maintain the glucose-insulin clamp and blood glucose rises into harmful territory. T2DM is not a disease of the pancreas, the pancreas is doing its genetically limited best, but it is a psychological disease of carbohydrate addiction where emotional management demands the consumption of massive quantities of sugar and starch far beyond the capacity of the pancreas to control.

Irrespective of genetic capacity to produce insulin, when chronic excessive carbohydrate consumption exceeds maximum insulin production over time, that difference is called T2DM. At first, doctors prescribe drugs that increase cellular sensitivity to glucose uptake, or flog the pancreas to super-increase insulin production, increase glucose removal from the bloodstream or increase glucose elimination in the urine, but eventually when even that fails, insulin itself is prescribed to cope with the amount of carbohydrate the patient is putting in their face. These drugs may lower the blood glucose number, but carbohydrates are toxic at ingestion. Lowering the numbers with exercise or medication only mildly reduces the harmful toxic effect the carbohydrates have on the body. The cause of T2DM is not a lack of insulin, it is a chronic excess of carbohydrate consumption that results in genetically predetermined failure of the insulin-glucagon blood glucose management system. Only the timing of onset of T2DM is affected by genetics, not whether or not someone is susceptible. Ironically, early onset of T2DM reduces the severity of obesity. Generally, the fatter a person is (another toxic consequence of chronic excessive carbohydrate consumption), the less likely they are to be diabetic because insulin drives sugar conversion to fat, but eventually everyone's pancreas will fail, weight gain slows, but T2DM ensues.

Type 1 Diabetes Mellitus

T1DM is a disease characterised by a lack of insulin production with disregulation of the insulin-glucagon blood glucose regulatory mechanism. These patients are typically on injectable insulin and are vulnerable to sugar highs (consumption-induced) and sugar lows (medication-induced). Because treatment is usually based on glycemic index principles, almost all T1DM have an additional Type 2 component added into the complexity of their disease. There is no reason a T1DM patient should not be managed according to carbohydrate abstinence principles. In our experience, this approach achieves the most sustained degree of tight glycemic control and the most effective way to stabilise medications at very basal levels. Glucagon production maintains adequate blood glucose levels between meals and insulin boluses are rarely required.

"Curing" T2DM

T2DM is not a blood glucose or insulin problem, T2DM is a substance abuse problem that results in end organ damage from toxic effects of chronic excessive carbohydrate consumption. Remission (normal diabetic indices and off medication) should be the goal of all T2DM treatment paradigms. To date, almost the entire paradigm of diabetic management is focused on lowering elevated blood glucose levels using sophisticated and very expensive drug regimens that, at best slow the progression of the disease without any form of remission. In fact, most practitioners do not believe in the concept of remission and believe T2DM is a chronic, relentless incurable disease that nearly always leads to morbidity and death. This misguided belief has spawned a whole industry dedicated to the treatment of diabetes-related co-morbidities and complications, the ramifications of which are likely to bankrupt most modern healthcare systems if left unresolved.

No surgeon would contemplate doing a liver transplant on an actively drinking alcoholic, yet that is essentially what every physician treating T2DM does with every prescription they write.

In order to set remission as a goal for our diabetic patients, we need to partner with them in the treatment process. Practitioner and patient should each clearly understand their roles. Effective treatment to the point of remission of any carbohydrate-induced CNCDs including T2DM requires a bimodal approach. Treat the cause and treat the disease.

Effective diabetic treatment requires a partnership between patient and physician. The physician's responsibility is to monitor and treat the diabetic numbers as well as complications and co-morbidities of the disease using appropriate medications or even surgery to reduce the impact of the disease. Philosophically, the intent should be to treat into remission, while being comfortable progressively withdrawing medication treatment as it becomes unnecessary, yet continuing to monitor for psychological relapse.

The patient's responsibility is to engage in a formal carbohydrate addiction cognitive behavioural modification therapy program ("Diabetic AA") to eliminate carbohydrate consumption inducing remission by abstaining from the use of sugar and moving toward an action-based endorphin release strategy while eating real food that does not contain carbohydrates.

Society's responsibility is to educate regarding the toxicity of carbohydrates and to regulate access and sale of carbohydrates in similar fashion to alcohol, nicotine and other psycho-active drugs including discouragement in the form of a "sin tax" the proceeds of which can assist in funding diabetic healthcare as we move to a universal healthcare system.

Remission requires application of physiologic as well as addiction principles. Physiologically, reducing the frequency and quantity of total carbohydrate consumption below the threshold of maximum insulin production allows the hepato-pancreatic glucagon-insulin feedback pathway to recover its control of carbohydrate metabolism thus preventing T2DM and putting it into remission where the blood glucose level is not causing harm. If we were rats in a cage and our access to carbohydrates was tightly controlled, such reduction in carbohydrate consumption could work.

However, by definition, by the time T2DM is measurable, the diabetic has lost control of their relationship with carbohydrates, and has become a carbohydrate addict. As with any other substance addiction, remission is only possible through abstinence because of the risk of return to excess in response to emotional distress. Reduction or modification of carbohydrate consumption may transiently improve the diabetic profile, but will not put it into remission, since with each unexpected emotional event, which is part of any diabetic's life, the dominant emotion-management strategy remains the carbohydrate high.

Successful treatment into remission requires Recognition, Removal and Replacement.

Recognition (and ownership of the problem)

Typically a person with T2DM consumes more than 75-90% of their total daily calories in the form of carbohydrates. The pattern of consumption is more like smoking than real meals. Not only is the total fraction of carbohydrate calories excessive, the pattern of consumption follows endorphin needs rather than somatic nutritional needs. Diabetics typically have more than 15-20 consumptive events per day, mostly in the form of carbohydrate snacks or drinks that pattern daily endorphin activation requirements. A snack is always an emotional event, never a nutritional event, and "hunger" is the need for an endorphin release through eating or drinking rather than a need to consume nutrients based on a somatic nutrient deficit.

Removal

Cognitive behavioural therapy for carbohydrate addicts begins with abstinence (see definition below) and removal of the drug from a patient's local environment. A return to nutritional eating rarely requires more than one or two eating events per day, breakfast being the least necessary. This is the divorce or deprivation phase. While carbohydrates are unnecessary for human survival, they do play two important, albeit dysfunctional roles in the addict's life, which are lost when the diabetic abstains from carbohydrates. First, because of the nutrient additives, they do provide some form of nutrition, enough to keep the diabetic alive, but not healthy or nutritionally replete. Diabetics are by definition malnourished. Secondly, carbohydrates are powerful endorphin activators, but function through the dysfunctional mechanisms of emotional repression, numbing and soothing rather than allowing processing and emotional therapy.

The word PERMISSION dominates addiction management. Removal requires internal cognitive wrestling with the distortion of reality whereby addicts give themselves permission to access their drug of choice despite knowledge of the consequences.

Replacement

In order to recover fully, patients need to replace carbohydrates with real food essential to healthy human existence using fat and protein as the primary macronutrients. They also need to change from an endorphin-based snacking eating pattern to a nutritional pattern, allowing the thirst and hunger centres to take back control of nutrition away from the endorphin centre. Humans typically require 1-3 nutritional events per day. More frequent consumptive events are for the mind not the body. While the body adapts to this new pattern of eating, keeping insulin levels basal allows the body to utilise circulating fat as the primary fuel source and ketosis is one of the most effective ways to suppress hunger. The fundamental concept is addiction not nutrition.

While abstinence is the goal, we limit our daily total carbohydrate consumption to <30 g total non-vegetable carbohydrates per day. This number helps conscious awareness of incidental carbohydrates like the 2 g of carbohydrate in the whole milk I use in my coffee. Unlike diets, it does not grant permission to consume carbohydrate dominant foods to make up to 30 g. Aside from rice and potato abstinence, using addiction principles, vegetables are free irrespective of their carbohydrate content because small amounts of carbohydrates found in vegetables do not have an endorphin-activating response and the nutrient value far exceeds the carbohydrate content. So, from a nutritional perspective, vegetables are free to eat, but not after "juicing" which is a method of extracting the drug from the food. After a rough stressful day, no person is reaching into the fridge for broccoli to soothe their mental anguish.

Secondly, replacement requires building up a repertoire of endorphin-alternatives. Preferably action-based rather than consumptive. It is common for smokers who successfully quit to gain weight. They are not quitting being addicts, they are merely doing a drug transfer from nicotine to carbohydrates. Successful endorphin replacement requires conscious forced engagement in doing little things on a regular basis as well as creating an action-based "fortress of solitude" where the person can escape to process their emotional needs until the new endorphin-releasing pattern becomes second nature.

Both patients and physicians need to be very aware that blood glucose levels may normalise very rapidly. If the patient abstains from carbohydrates, but continues to take their diabetic medication, they may induce hypoglycemia. Ironically, most physicians who treat diabetics ask them to consume carbohydrates to elevate their blood sugar rather than reducing their medication. When working toward remission, the opposite needs to happen. Close monitoring of blood glucose levels during this time is critical. With the assumption that the diabetic is conforming to carbohydrate abstinence principles and is not snacking, we use a fasting blood glucose of 140 mg/dL as a guide. If the blood glucose level is at or below this number, we halve the medication or insulin daily until it is no longer taken. If the blood glucose level rebounds above 160 mg/dL we add a third of the medication back, but also ask the patient to review what they consumed. In our experience, most Type 2 diabetics are able to come off their medication with normal blood glucose levels (our definition of remission) within 2-4 weeks of starting the protocol. C-peptide and insulin levels may remain elevated longer as a reflection of insulin resistance. Under these circumstances, we leave our patients on small doses of metformin until their insulin-based glucagon suppression returns. HbA1c levels come down slower as glycosylated red blood cells get replaced with normal ones, with an expectation of HbA1c<5.4 by one year in those successfully abstaining from carbohydrates.

The reason we cannot use the word CURE, despite normalisation of diabetic parameters, is because addictions are chronically relapsing disorders and maintenance is critical. Relapses happen and while a relapse needs to be treated cognitively, the astute physician should also be observant for a trend toward T2DM once again. While the disease needs to be treated medically, the threat of recurrence may be a powerful tool to induce abstinence again.

There are no powders or potions, shakes or shots, pills, gimmicks, gadgets or surgeries that can treat the addiction. The only effective medication is salt water – sweat, tears and maybe a walk beside the ocean.

Summary

Numbers do not cause disease and all because the diabetic numbers are below a treatment threshold, it does not mean that harmful diabetogenic pathology is not occurring. Diabetogenesis is the toxicity mediated by chronic excessive carbohydrate consumption irrespective of whether the blood glucose numbers meet a treatment threshold. As physicians we need to be as concerned about diabetogenesis as we are about diabetes.

Carbohydrates are as powerfully psychoactive as nicotine, alcohol and opioids, and are as rapidly addictive. Unless you are a performance athlete, most Type 2 diabetics are simply people who over time have transitioned away from eating for the nutritional value of food toward eating primarily for the endorphin release and emotional management effect of a powerful psychoactive drug called sugar.

Carbohydrates help us to soothe and numb the entire spectrum of our emotional needs (stress, anxiety, depression, boredom, pleasure, etc.) When our relationship with carbohydrates becomes the dominant, if not exclusive way in which we absolve our emotional needs, over time, harm happens including T2DM, obesity, hypertension, dyslipidemia, sleep apnea, polycystic ovarian syndrome and most of the other metabolic CNCDs. When we distort the reality of this harm and continue the relationship with sugar, we lose control of the relationship. This is addiction.

Despite spending billions of dollars on trying to understand and treat the complex pathophysiology of T2DM and other CNCDs, we are losing the battle for one simple reason – we have yet to understand, let alone acknowledge, that T2DM, obesity and the associated CNCDs are quite simply a substance abuse problem directly caused by uncontrolled chronic excessive carbohydrate consumption – carbohydrate abuse and addiction. No sugar, no disease. How much harm did we suffer as a society until we restricted and controlled alcohol and nicotine? How long will it take us, how threatened does our survival as a species need to become before we begin to regulate sugar?

The epidemic of T2DM and obesity is just another chapter following that of alcoholism a century ago, requiring Prohibition in the USA to stem the epidemic, followed by smoking fifty years ago and just now beginning to wane. The same vulnerable population has merely done a substance transfer from alcohol to nicotine to carbohydrates. Understanding the epidemiology of these addiction epidemics and the nature of addiction rather than addressing a particular substance issue will be the best defense in the protection of future generations from the scourge of addiction.

Post Script: our results

Clinical data in support of a carbohydrate addiction cognitive behavioural treatment program

Since 2003, we have run a bariatric practice founded on the premise that obesity and related co-morbid illnesses are a direct consequence of chronic excessive carbohydrate consumption.[5] We have used a carbohydrate addiction cognitive behavioural therapeutic model as the basis of our treatment algorithm using the concepts of Prochaska's "Changing for Good"[6] and a modified 12 step-type program similar to that used by Alcoholics Anonymous. We promote a return to nutritional eating using Low-Carb-High-Fat (LCHF) principles and we use bariatric surgery (intragastric balloons, gastric banding and sleeve gastrectomy) when needed as tools to assist patients in dealing with their carbohydrate addiction. As a clinical program, with over 800,000 personal treatment contacts with this population over the past 18 years, we have a vast experience and a wealth of anecdotal data, however, a paucity of prospective scientific study data. A particular focus has been our adolescent carbohydrate addiction management program and below we present summary results of a three year retrospective analysis of our data in this population.[7]

Children & adolescents

The presence of adverse health conditions such as T2DM, hypertension, and dyslipidemia occurring in conjunction with childhood obesity is well documented in the literature, but these conditions are often under-diagnosed in children. Adolescents have a better chance of resolving hyperinsulinemia compared to adults.[8]

We conducted a retrospective single arm data analysis to determine the proportion of obese adolescents between the ages of 10-20 years, who had undiagnosed co-morbidities upon initial evaluation at our medical clinic specialising in the treatment of severe obesity and related health conditions. The data set includes all patients, aged 10-20 years, diagnosed as obese and who had been tested at intake for T2DM, hypertension, and dyslipidemia from 2010-2012. The study population size was n=110. At intake, two categories for co-morbidities, a) prior history and b) diagnosis at intake, were created in the data set in order to determine the amount of previously undiagnosed co-morbidities. We then treated this cohort over a three-year period using carbohydrate addiction cognitive behavioural therapy together with gastric banding surgery.

Since 2010, the American Diabetes Association[9] has recommended the use of the HbA1c test to diagnose diabetes in adults, with a threshold of ≥6.5%.[10, 11] However, there are no percentile charts for diagnosis or treatment of T2DM in children.[12] Several prospective studies that used HbA1c to predict the progression to diabetes demonstrated a strong, continuous association between HbA1c and subsequent diabetes. In a systematic review of 44,203 individuals from 16 cohort studies with a follow-up interval averaging 5.6 years (range 2.8–12 years), those with an HbA1c between 5.5 and 6.0% had a substantially increased risk of diabetes with 5-year incidences ranging from 9 to 25%. An HbA1c range of 6.0–6.5% had a 5-year risk of developing diabetes between 25 to 50% and relative risk (RR) 20 times higher compared with an HbA1c of 5.0%.[13] Baseline HbA1c was a stronger predictor of subsequent diabetes and cardiovascular events than was fasting glucose.[14]

Therefore, it is reasonable to consider an HbA1c range of 5.7–6.4% as identifying individuals with pre-diabetes. As with glucose measurements, the continuum of risk is curvilinear, so that as HbA1c rises, the risk of diabetes rises disproportionately.[15] Accordingly, interventions should be most intensive and follow-up particularly vigilant for those with HbA1c above 6.0%, who should be considered to be at very high risk. Given this information, we set the threshold for the diagnosis in our adolescent at an HbA1c >6.0%.

For the diagnosis of T2DM, we measure HbA1c, C-peptide, insulin and fasting blood glucose.

Table 1 shows the socio-demographic characteristics of the study population. The mean age for this 10 to 20 year old cohort was 16.4 years and the median age was 16.0 years. All subjects in this study were diagnosed as morbidly obese (CDC table Body Mass Index (kg/m^2) >97th percentile for age) at the intake evaluation, with a mean BMI of 46.1 kg/m^2 and a median BMI of 44.2 kg/m^2. After an average of 22 months from the intake evaluation, with subsequent bariatric surgery and peri-operative carbohydrate addiction cognitive behavioural therapy with a goal of carbohydrate abstinence (<30 g non-vegetable total carbohydrate consumption per day), the mean BMI for this cohort was 29.8 kg/m^2 and the median BMI was 29.1 kg/m^2.

TABLE 1 Sociodemographic Characteristics of the Study Population

Characteristics	N (unweighted)	Percentage (unweighted)
Sex	110	
Males	42	38.2
Females	68	61.8
Race	110	
White	58	52.7
Black	36	32.7
Hispanic/other	16	14.6
Continuous Variables	**Mean**	**Median**
Age	16.4 years	16.0 years
Initial BMI	46.1 kg/m^2	44.2 kg/m^2
Final BMI	29.8 kg/m^2	29.1 kg/m^2

Findings from the statistical analyses of co-morbidity prevalence in this study population are summarised in Table 2.

TABLE 2 **Prevalence of Comorbidities in Study Population**

Variables		Percentage
Type 2 diabetes	History prior to initial evaluation	15.5
	Diagnosis	28.0
	After 22 months treatment	7.2
Dyslipidemia	History prior to initial evaluation	8.2
	Diagnosis	30.7
	After 22 months treatment	12.7

At intake evaluation, 15.5% (n=17) of patients had a history of T2DM on medication. Among those patients who did not have a history of T2DM at intake evaluation (n=93), data analysis showed that 28.0% (n=26) were newly diagnosed, prior to treatment, as having T2DM. Therefore, in this study population a total of 39.1% (n=43) patients had a HbA1c>6.0%. After 22 months of treatment, 7.2% (n=8) still met our criteria for T2DM and 4.5% (n=5) remained on at least 1 diabetic medication. Of the patients that had T2DM at the end of the study period, none had successfully sustained carbohydrate abstinence and all had at least one additional significant co-morbidity (obesity, hypertension or dyslipidemia). At the intake evaluation, 11.8% (n=13) of patients had a history of hypertension (>140/90 mmHg for subjects 14 to 20 years of age; for subjects under 14 years of age, BP> 97th percentile for age). Among those patients who did not have a history of hypertension at intake evaluation (n=97), data analysis showed that 42.3% (n=41) were newly diagnosed prior to treatment, as having hypertension. After 22 months of treatment, 6.4% (n=7) still had hypertension but none were on medication. At intake evaluation, 8.2% (n=9) of patients had a history of dyslipidemia (having any one of the following, 1) total cholesterol greater than 200 mg/dL, 2) LDL greater than 100 mg/dL, 3) HDL-C less than 39 mg/dL, or 4) triglyceride level greater than 150 mg/dL). Among those patients who did not have a history of dyslipidemia at intake evaluation (n=101), data analysis showed that 30.7% (n=31) were newly diagnosed prior to treatment, as having dyslipidemia. After 22 months of treatment, 12.7% (n=14) had dyslipidemia.

Of note is that, during the time of this study, our diet modification was primarily focused on carbohydrate abstinence (<30 g non-vegetable total carbohydrate consumption per day) with an increase in protein as the alternative macronutrient. Based on these data and the evidence in support of a high fat diet as documented elsewhere in this book, we have since implemented an LCHF protocol. Anecdotally, we have seen further improvements in co-morbid parameters, but more importantly, once patients become fat-adapted, it appears that there is greater appetite suppression and sustainability of the diet with fewer relapse episodes.

A note on surgery for T2DM

Without adequate or substantive long term data, there has been a trend within the bariatric surgical community to view surgery as a "cure" for T2DM.[16] There is no question that bariatric surgery does reduce the severity of T2DM for a period of time. This clearly benefits the patient, but is the long term risk of surgery less than the ultimate risk of the improvement in diabetes numbers? Most recently, based upon evidence of transient normalisation of diabetic numbers, bariatric surgeons have proclaimed that Roux-en-Y Gastric Bypass surgery and duodenal switch surgery "cures" diabetes. No operation on the stomach cures the head. It is true that by altering the hunger-satiety feedback pathways and the site and rate of absorption of carbohydrates, as well as the glycemic index of sugars consumed, there is a transient reduction in frequency as well as quantity of carbohydrate consumption that improves the diabetic numbers, even into normal range. But diabetes is not a number, it is a vascular disease process mediated by a drug called sugar, and to proclaim an addict "cured" is naive and irresponsible without adequate supportive data. All because an alcoholic's blood alcohol level is 0.07 g/dL, and they are below the DUI threshold of 0.08 g/dL it may mean they will not get arrested, but it does not mean that they are safe to drive or sober. If their blood alcohol level is frequently elevated, but they are not drunk, it does not mean they will not get liver disease.

The effective durability of bariatric surgery in terms of an ongoing positive weight loss response is no more than 1-3 years, after which the surgery is no longer effective in inducing change. Either the patient has used their surgery as a tool to help them address their addiction, and their diabetes stays in remission because of their change in carbohydrate consumption, or the disease insidiously returns along with malnutrition, weight and co-morbidity regain. Based upon our experience, despite excellent initial weight loss and co-morbidity resolution, but because of the high prevalence of subsequent complications including surgical as well as metabolic and malnutrition, I do not believe that the Roux-en-y gastric bypass or the duodenal switch or any other primarily malabsorbtive procedure should be performed as a first line surgery in humans – especially in the era of sleeve gastrectomy and gastric banding. Initially, the body may seem to compensate very effectively to malabsorbtive operations, and the reduction in weight and co-morbidities in response to "comfortable starvation" seem to be miraculous, but the body has to be getting its nutrients from somewhere. Typically, this is from its own stores that are plentiful enough to sustain the patient for up to a few years before the deficiencies become clinically detectable to the astute physician. Who is going to notice a 50% demineralisation of the skeleton over 10 years? But most of these storage depletions are irrecoverable and the bariatric patient pays a malnutrition price for their thinness.

While I do advocate for restrictive-type bariatric surgery as a life-saving tool to be used in carefully selected cases to help patients deal with their addiction, to market surgery as a magical cure is highly irresponsible, dangerous and in my opinion, malpractice.

Dr Robert Cywes

Case Study: Indya

Florida-born Indya was always an overweight child. But then it crept up and up during her teens. She celebrated her 20th birthday in hospital, bedridden, weighting 600 lbs and suffering a host of health issues. As she was lying in an intensive care bed, unable to breathe for herself, she decided that it was time for a life or death decision.
She chose life, and started her amazing journey back to health.

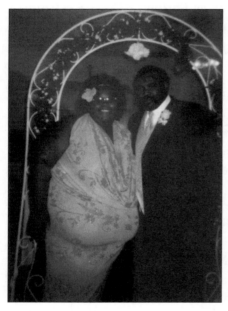

As a bedridden teenager, I saw the bleakest of futures. Now I am 32, enjoying life, and am an inspiring recording artist. Home in a condo near the beach with my wonderful brother in Jacksonville, Florida.

Looking back, I was always an overweight child, but never really thought about the health problems. I spent my teenage years being very active in high school – from student body president and JROTC to Ladies of Raines and other various prestigious clubs. This all culminated in a full-paid scholarship to the University of North Florida.

However, the dream was about to come crashing down.

Throughout high school, my weight was going up and up. Healthy eating was rarely encouraged, and all my group activities in school kept me socially-accepted by my peers.

I eventually came to the conclusion, over time, that I had an addiction to food; and as time went on my weight began to pile on. 300 lbs. 400 lbs. 500 lbs.

My weight affected everything in my life. Months after I arrived at college, it seemed like everything turned for the worse. I was either ill or had no energy. I couldn't get up in the morning, so was missing classes.

I starved myself, but continued to gain weight drastically, with no explanation as to why.

The mystery started to unravel when a cut on my leg would not stop leaking water for days. I was rushed to hospital, where I was told that I was suffering from Edema, which caused my body to retain water causing weight gain.

The excess fluid then started to cover my heart and lungs.

I was still a teenager, at college, and was supposed to be experiencing the best days of my life. Yet at 19, I was bedridden, requiring oxygen, with Congestive Heart Failure, Diabetes, Chronic Asthma, Sleep Apnea, Edema, Bronchitis, and all the aches and pains you could imagine.

The scales topped out at 600 lbs and I was also battling mental depression.

And things got really bad.

I was 'celebrating' my 20th birthday in the intensive care unit and overheard the doctor ask my mother about hospice arrangements. I felt helpless. I was unable to breathe on my own, needed others to wheel me around, and now my mortality was on the agenda.

That was it. I had a life I wanted to live, so I chose to fight back and live. But how?

That answer came in the form of a ray of sunshine called Dr Robert Cywes. He opened my eyes to the fact that the foods I loved were destroying my life.

I wanted gastric surgery, but had to lose 150 lbs beforehand. The low-carb lifestyle Dr Cywes offered would feed my body what it really needed and help me reach, then smash, that magic figure.

Dr Cywes and his team would also offer me the tools, knowledge and motivation I would need to make that life change.

Together with my low-carb diet, I started exercising from my wheelchair and my bed. Once I built enough strength, I started pushing my wheelchair and oxygen tank around my bedroom, then the living room, and then I made it outside.

I never allowed the sniggers and stares to deter me, because I had a bigger vision in mind.

A combination of my low-carb food and water tablets worked wonders. The weight started to come off and I no longer needed to carry oxygen everywhere I went. I no longer had to worry for my life when my oxygen tank ran low.

The small things we take for granted like BREATHING!

I moved on to exercising in a swimming pool and aerobics.

I lost 190 lbs, was able to get lap band surgery, and then lost an additional 150 lbs.

I did fall off the wagon at some stage, when my craving for carbohydrates reared its ugly head. Before I knew it, I had gained more than 50 lbs, but Dr Cywes came to my rescue again.

He got me back on track mentally, and with some additional gastric surgery, my low carb diet and plenty of exercise have worked wonders.

Any medications and oxygen support are in the past, and I've lost more than two-thirds of my body weight. Yes, I am so proud to announce that I am down to 180 lbs!

My life has drastically changed and I feel like I can live again. Never in a million years did I see myself able to zip line, go para-sailing, or just experience the simple joy of amusement park rides.

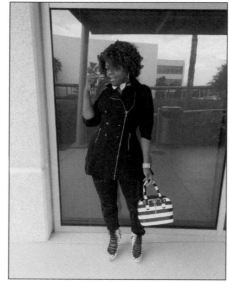

I am proud to announce I went from 'wheels to heels', and I am thankful for the gift of life. I embrace every moment of it.

My advice to anyone currently struggling with diabetes is that you should embrace life too. In order to succeed in anything, you must at first try. Never allow the fear of failure take over. The battle is yours to win.

The different types

Chapter Five

How a Type 1 diabetic doctor runs half marathons on a ketogenic diet

Dr Ian Lake

I dodged a bullet on the day I discovered the ketogenic diet. It was a shift in my knowledge that transformed my life. I have discovered so much in the last couple of years that I cannot begin to believe how I could have thought otherwise. I have Type 1 Diabetes and am also a GP. So I am talking Type 1 from both sides of the consulting desk.

National guidelines currently cling onto the belief that a healthy, balanced diet must contain a lot of carbohydrate and not a lot of fat. But the evidence is suggesting that this is not the case at all. The reverse is likely to be true, more fats from real food sources and restricted carbohydrates.

Slightly more troubling is the notion that the high carbohydrate model can be extended to diabetes, which is a condition of carbohydrate intolerance. If you have a carbohydrate intolerant body, why on earth would you feed it carbohydrates? Most of the old school would reply with 'because it is a major food group and is essential' (which of course it isn't) as if it was as obvious as the fact that the sun goes round the earth. But now there is new thinking on this which is getting good results. A paradigm shift is imminent. But the old paradigm has dug its heels in. Big time. Some influential scientists have made the age-old mistake of seeing their speciality as a fact, not a current best-fit, and have become high priests of their own quasi-religions. Business has of course moved in to exploit an opportunity. As long as the old paradigm can be propped up, that will be the case. But in the end the new paradigm will replace the old one. It is the order of things.

This paradigm shift will be a change of consensus from the ground up. The internet has linked people up like never before. Everyone can now access the same information that was previously only available to those in power. People can spread the message. Slowly, the old paradigm will lose its power, not because of some winner-takes-all battle, but because it will become irrelevant.

So, what's my contribution to the revolution? Well, by using my status as both a patient and a doctor, I can show that some of the current beliefs on diet in diabetes have no foundation at all. I decided to set out to prove beyond all doubt that carbohydrates are not essential in Type 1 Diabetes, and that a ketogenic diet is a safe option for exercise. It is the ignorant perpetuation of the insulin-carbohydrate model that really gets me going. So I have undertaken a series of monthly half marathons to explore ketogenic diets and fasting in Type 1 Diabetes: 12 half marathons in 12 months, to be precise. I have passed on the information in a blog (www.type1keto.com) and I think that I have proven my case. If the insulin dose is correct, then carbs are not necessary in Type 1 Diabetes. I am still here. I have proved what I set out to test and learned so much along the way. I am healthier, and, for the first time in years, optimistic about my diabetic future. I have a normal HbA1c for the first time in two decades.

This project started out as a test of what I thought was 'extreme' diabetes, as it was way outside of the current guidelines. I even blogged as "Lemming Test-Pilot", as that's what I felt like – a lemming leaping over the edge of the cliff into the unknown. I now realise that the real 'extreme' diabetes is trying to run following the Insulin-Carb model. I really do take my hat off to those guys. They are taking huge risks compared to me.

Me and my diabetes

I have Type 1 diabetes and have had it for 20 years. I got it relatively late, in my 30s. My blood pressure is okay, and my cholesterol in the 5s. I have tried hard to manage my diabetes in the conventional way. 55% carbs, 30% fat mostly unsaturated, basal (long acting) insulin, and DAFNE (Dose Adjustment For Normal Eating) with carbohydrate counting and injection of rapid acting insulin to balance the glucose. I look after my weight, and exercise regularly. I have tried three types of statins at various doses, but had to stop due to muscle pains and fatigue. I try to look after my condition to the best of my ability and have been following the NICE (National Institute for Care and Health

98

Excellence) guidelines. I regularly attend check-ups. My GP or Diabetes Nurse takes my measurements every year, makes some suggestions for improvement (there is always room for improvement!), then leaves me to it for another year. My GP team manage me 0.2% of the year. I manage myself 99.8%.

Unless they have diabetes, or are close to someone who has, clinicians would find it difficult to imagine what us diabetics go through on a daily basis. For example: forgetting if we have taken our insulin doses; running out of supplies; eating out and forgetting insulin, or worse, injecting early and the food arrives late; feeling hypo and having no glucose; just not feeling right and wondering if it is due to glucose or not; being drunk and not knowing if the morning after is a hypo or hangover; re-using needles or injecting through clothes to be discrete. Life as a diabetic is a constant struggle, trying to master the almost impossible dark art of carbohydrate counting and medication balance. Mini-hypos are not uncommon, but dangerous ones are rare. I have had hypos regularly for 20 years, but I've only been caught out twice, when I needed help, and both were due to my stupidity. My medical team are really good and seem to understand me well. They have been looking after me for 20 years and I think the continuity of care has helped a lot.

However, despite some of the best medical care in the world, I was not doing as well as I would have liked. My HbA1c was creeping up and my insulin doses were increasing. The thing was though, it really was not lack of effort. But the nuancing of the advice in my medical consultation made me think it might be. Was I simply not trying hard enough, (or was that just my paranoia)? No, I am beginning to understand that I personally have been on the wrong diet. And have been for 20 years! Any other condition managed with the wrong treatment for 20 years would rightly merit a lawsuit. The guideline advisers are getting knighthoods!

I finally got round to implementing something I had read about only as recently as 2015. You see, I was getting desperate. I had had a few hypo crises, slightly more unannounced than before. Not unmanageable, but I was needing to be more careful. They were a brooding shadow over my outdoor active lifestyle. And, worse, I was feeling old, with joint aches, general stiffness, often fogged thought and disabling dizzy spells when I stood up from sitting. Nothing specific, just below what I felt should be normal. I was also injecting higher doses of insulin with no improvement in control. Not a good place to be.

I turned to a ketogenic diet as a last throw of the dice, but it was difficult to reject the advice on fats and carbs that I had believed in for the previous 20 years of diabetes. The medical world in which I work is completely integrated with the official 'healthy eating' messages. We have taken on board the whole lexicon of the advertising industry with 'healthy' grains, 'complex' carbs, 'low-fat' and the like. We are where we are and where we are is in a total mess! I suppose that insulin is a convenient tool to counter the carbs, so the 'healthy, balanced' (advertising again), diet has just been extended to diabetes.

Well, for me I can say definitely that this is wrong. I have done just about everything to improve carbohydrate and insulin balance, eaten all of the 'healthy balanced' foods for 20 years. In just one year, doing almost exactly the opposite, I am in control and healthy. For the first time since the diagnosis of my "lifelong, disabling" condition, I feel that I might have a chance...

Assessing the risks

Balancing insulin and carbohydrate is fundamental to managing Type 1 Diabetes. The position statement from the American Diabetes Association is quite clear on carb counting in management and the level of evidence, level B, is impressive: "Monitoring carbohydrate intake, whether by carbohydrate counting or experience-based estimation, remains a key strategy in achieving glycaemic control".

Quite right. If you are eating carbohydrate and have diabetes it is definitely a good idea to monitor it! But there is no research that I can find in the guidelines that has looked at carbohydrate and insulin with respect to whether you *need* carbohydrate...

I had been advised to manage my diabetes by injecting extra insulin, rapid-acting, at mealtimes depending on how many carbohydrate portions I had consumed. That is standard carbohydrate counting and insulin management, with which we diabetics are all very familiar. But, if we eat no carbs with meals, how much extra insulin do we then need? Well, the answer is none, surely. No extra insulin beyond background. If your meal carbohydrate count is zero, the required insulin is then zero... is that the case? I realised that eating carbs, as a diabetic, just didn't make sense. I was completely unaware of any research looking at, say, a diet of 10% carbohydrate and 75% fat – not 55% carb and 30% fat. It left me thinking that I had received 20 years of dietary advice that just didn't apply to me.

A half marathon with problems

As I explained above, living as a diabetic (either type to be honest) is difficult enough – living as an active diabetic, who enjoys exercise, provides another challenge on top. I woke on the morning I was due to run a half marathon wondering what should I inject for this run? I need about 10 units of long-acting insulin twice a day; occasionally less, but only by a couple of units or so. That is my reliable basal dose. Blood glucose at breakfast that morning was 5.4 mmol/l, with no sign of a dawn phenomenon. This was very strange. In fact I had a fairly flat trace that morning, which was not typical. But diabetes throws up things like that from time to time. The key to success is being able to adapt. It would have been tempting to ignore the rapid-acting insulin. I had just eaten a keto breakfast. But the sausage did look dodgy in respect to carbs. Also in my experience there would be the glucose raising effect of the adrenaline during the race. I would likely be going above 7 mmol/l at some point in the next couple of hours from experience. So, I decided to inject two units of rapid-acting insulin. This was an hour and a half before the run. I know that my rapid-acting insulin is just not that. Not rapid at all. More like three hours, so its effect would be peaking in the last part of the run.

The action of insulin is predictable in each individual. Mine starts acting at 3 hours then reduces glucose by 6 mmol/l per hour for the next 3 hours. I know that 1 unit of insulin reduces my glucose by 2.2 mmols/l.[1] So 2 units of insulin gives a 4.4 mmol/l reduction in glucose (plus a bit more for the long acting but negligible over an hour or so). The rate of reduction of 6 mmols/l/hour means that those 2 units would produce a 4 mmol/l reduction in blood glucose over the period of 40 minutes or so that I would expect to be running with rapid-acting insulin working. Therefore, a glucose of 8 mmol/l at one and a half hours running would get me to about 3.6 by the end of the run. I reckoned I would go with that, factoring in the adrenaline of the run and the protein in the bacon. And goodness knows what was in the sausage. It was all educated guesswork anyway. Give it a go! With no carbs to interfere, calculations were relatively easy. But this run was not as planned. It was the failure of the dawn phenomenon which caught me out. I went low at about half way and needed about 20 g of carbs to rescue the situation. But overall it was encouraging. Before I decided to choose a ketogenic diet, I would never have contemplated doing a second long run, after the previous one a month earlier. I don't think I could have done it. So that was good. But clearly I had used too much insulin at some point. Possibly I did more activity before the run because we needed to walk a fair way to get to the venue. It was disappointing to need carbs to rescue the situation. I was trying to do these runs purely on keto after all. But it was only the second event. Safety is always paramount. I carried glucose for that reason. It is difficult to finish a run when unconscious through a hypo. So a certain amount of flexibility is prudent and practical.

A half marathon with ketogenic support

I read somewhere recently that a sign of high intelligence is learning from one's mistakes. Well that makes me Stephen Hawking! Probably most diabetics fall into that camp – because we simply have to learn from mistakes or we can end up in big trouble. I learned from the previous run. Big time. I was also over-training for my fitness level, so I decided to give the rest of the week a miss and 'wing it'. Winging it has been my modus operandi of life and has worked so far. So, wing-it it was. The last half-marathon was the second half-marathon in two months that I had done. That was already new ground for me, so this third one was completely uncharted territory. All this talk of uncharted territory and the like is a mental thing, I guess. In reality a half-marathon is a completely manageable couple of hours running. And nothing more. I guess we are all limited by our own sense of what is possible

Challenging oneself is exciting. I have done my fair share of risky things in adventure sports over the years. The dare, the apprehension, the decision to commit and the adrenaline rush are addictive. In adventure sports, other brave people have 'been there' before and have learned from mistakes to improve safety. All I have to do is to do what I am told by my instructor, and be taught how to assess the risk. Then do it.

In this series of experiments with diabetes, I was constantly warned that what I was attempting to do was against all scientific consensus. In its own way, stepping outside the norm of medical practice is just as daunting as risk sports. If not more so. There are of course pioneers in the field of ketogenic diets who have laid the groundwork. I am grateful and was keen to use that experience to the full.[2] But I felt sure that my guideline diet of high carbohydrate and low fat had brought me to the brink of a personal health disaster. So, with risk sports, whereas you make a positive decision to *take the risk*, with these experiments I made a positive decision to *reduce* the risk. The short-term experiments, like this series of runs, were a challenge, but I was pretty sure I had a sound knowledge of the biochemistry, and that they would work. Risky, possibly, but I was sure that the gains would be found in the longer term. The experts will tell you that it is risky. They'll tell you that there is little evidence for the benefits of keto in the longer term. I came to the conclusion that the biggest risk I could take would be to continue to do the same thing that I had been doing for 20 years. I was just declining in health by doing that. Ironically there is plenty of good evidence to say that decline in health will happen with diabetes – it just seems to be accepted. Doing the same thing over and over and expecting different results seemed doomed to fail. Ask Einstein. He defined insanity like that…. So, there came a point when I decided I had to look beyond what I had been told was normal. My new normal would be what I previously thought as not possible.

On the next half marathon at the one hour mark, about half way, my blood glucose peaked at a way too high 13 mmol/l. Then it started to fall at a predictable rapid insulin rate of 6 mmol/l per hour. So, I reckoned that, with one hour left to run, I would finish with a glucose level of seven or so. That was the theory and that is what happened. I took slightly longer to run the distance and the final glucose was just under this. But it all worked out. The small insulin doses turned out to work well. I just felt safe. At less than half way into a run I could totally relax and ignore my diabetes. I could think about something else. What a luxury that is. If you have Type 1 you will connect with this. It can be difficult to remember forgetting diabetes.

So what was my learning this time? I had done well. I had made progress. I had completed a half-marathon carbohydrate free and with reasonable glucose control. I learned that the practice of injecting insulin and not covering with carbs can be done. I learned that I was starting to love the keto diet!

A half marathon on fat

Having run the last half-marathon without carbs, I decided to try one fuelling on fat. Clearly I wanted to choose healthy fat, so that needed to be fat from pasture grazed animals, or oil processed by pressing with no industrial processes. I decided to go for coconut oil and unsalted butter. I have found a recipe for Bulletproof Coffee. Well a derivative of that: double strength coffee, 30 g of coconut oil and 20 g of butter, whisked up. Coconut oil is 87% sat fat (the rest is unsaturated fat and it has 860 calories per 100 g.[3] Butter has 717 calories per 100 g. It is 81% fat (the rest is water and a trace of carbohydrate and protein. The 81 g of fat per 100 g of butter comprises 51 g saturated and the rest is unsaturated.[4] (When people tell you that butter is saturated fat – they're only half right! My Bulletproof Coffee thus delivers a total of 400 calories, all as fat, which seems to be just what the doctor ordered for a run. I reserved the right to add some fibre if I felt sick! I allowed my body to provide the rest of the energy I needed, which I estimated to be about 100 g (3.5 oz of body fat. I could give that up okay.

On the morning of this run, I woke with a glucose approaching 7 mmol/l and allowed myself just one unit of insulin rapid-acting to nudge the glucose down a couple of mmol/l. Remember that one unit of insulin in someone of my weight (75 kg reduces glucose by 2.2 mmol/l. I used the same amount of long acting insulin, 10 units. That is my reliable dose. And I drank a glass of 300 ml plain water....

I arrived one hour before the run, so I brewed up the coffee in the car park and blended it with the pre-weighed 30 g coconut oil and 20 g butter. A vigorous shake and it was done. A creamy, greasy, black mix. It tasted quite reasonable. Oily on the palate, but the coffee and coconut came through strongly with notes of butter following. For fluid intake, I have found 4-500 ml per hour works well in normal UK conditions, so I consumed another 250 ml fluid as plain coffee, meeting half my needs well in advance.

My blood glucose level was 6.3 mmol/l in the 20 minutes before the run. At the half way point it was approaching 7 mmol, which was good and bang on the prediction. My time was good at seven miles – more encouragement. There were plenty of hills, which I had not expected (that means 'had not allowed for' being a diabetic). The glucometer sensor fell off at the 8 mile mark with a glucose of 7.3 mmol/l, but I felt good. I could stop worrying about a hypo. One unit of rapid acting was not going to do much. The main concern at this point was, had I injected *enough* insulin?

With enough insulin, everything is fine. Regulated fat burning, normal, healthy levels of ketones and business as usual with normal glucose levels. The ketogenic diet is safe in Type 1 diabetes, if one injects sufficient insulin.

It turned out that I had, indeed, injected enough insulin. I had a glucose reading of 3.9 mmol/l just after the run. It was vindication of the theory that you can inject insulin and not need carbs if you plan it properly.

My learning on this run was that I had demonstrated that basal insulin is sufficient to meet the metabolic needs of the body during a two hour period of moderate intensity exercise, fuelling on fat and when no carbohydrate is eaten. And beyond as well. Because after the run it was completely stable between 4 mmol/l and 7 mmol/l through the night and into the morning.

So, there you have it. If you don't eat carbs, you don't need extra insulin. What I had thought all along....

A half marathon on fast!

I had proven that a Type 1 diabetic (me anyway) could run for approximately two hours without any carbohydrate at all. That got me thinking. If I can do a half-marathon using dietary fat (coconut oil and butter) and some body fat, could I run the full distance on just body fat? (I told you I liked a challenge!)

I estimated that I would need approximately 1,200 calories. Body fat can supply approximately 7000 calories per kg, so 1200 calories is around 170 g. Nothing in the grand scheme of things. After all what exactly is a 'fast'? If we eat say, a couple of hours before a run, does that make the following couple of hours of not eating a 'fast'? The body will need to get its energy from somewhere in that time. 'It will get that energy from food', you say. Possibly, and ultimately yes. But it has to be processed first. So, yes, you need energy, of course you do. But it is also true that most of us have enough energy already stored as body fat. I know I have. Even though I am right in the middle of the range of BMI, I have some spare fat. I can see it. Just a hint of a wobble in the mirror. But it is there.

So I planned to do a 13 hour fast. There was no science in this amount of time. 13 hours and 13 miles had a catchy ring to it. Nothing more than that. 13 hours of not eating. All that would happen would be that I would slowly burn fat. Slowly during the fast, and then more quickly during the run. Increase the energy and use the same fuel. But burn at a slightly faster rate. I am a slow runner in the grand scheme of things. Olympians might take a different view and prepare differently. But I reckon that I represent the majority of runners. So, just let the fat burn: that seemed totally logical to me. It was quite exciting really, a bit of a leap into the unknown.

In fact simple fasting was to be a good strategy for this run as the organisers had cocked-up the parking arrangements. It was a fraught time getting to the start. We had to abandon the car and run two miles to the start line. I had injected the usual reliable 10 units of long- acting insulin on waking. In the hour before the run I was so pre-occupied with actually getting to the start that I forgot to manage the rapid- acting insulin. That mostly means, should I inject or not? When we arrived at the venue my continuous glucose meter was showing 6 mmol/l and a relatively flat trace. The glucose level had not gone up significantly during the two mile dash to the start, so possibly wouldn't. I always expect a bit of a spike in the mornings and usually shoot up a couple of units of rapid-acting on waking. I had not done that for this run because of the circumstances. So, what to do with the rapid acting? One unit of insulin reduces glucose by 2.2 mmol/l. Could I risk dropping any further from 6 mmol/l? Possibly the long acting would be cutting in right at the end as well. It usually just keeps the glucose levels flat but can dip throughout the day at a very slow rate. Not a big issue generally but it might be in this run. In the end I went with one unit. That would take the glucose down to somewhere just under four towards the end of the run. Note how scientific this wasn't. It was educated guesswork. I was rushing. Things go wrong when rushing. I had decided to take my rapid-acting pen with me just in case the glucose went up. I had an idea it wouldn't, but I was unsure. But, having grabbed a pen from my bag to take with me, I had forgotten the needle! So it was a couple of hundred metres run back to the bag drop building. Of course the needle was not in the bag (it was later found on the floor of the car). But luckily the long-acting pen was there. So I unscrewed the needle from the long-acting pen and used that. Just another day in the life of a person with diabetes!

Once settled in, the run itself was enjoyable. I had good energy levels, and with someone to talk to throughout, the miles just reeled away. Glucose levels were okay up to about an hour and a half when the blood glucose trickled down to 3.5 mmol/l at 10 miles. I became aware of a hypo just before the continuous glucose monitor squawked to tell me so. It was no big deal, just an increased sense of exhaustion really. Over the next mile I used 15 g of glucose tablets to top up. No drama at all. I opted to walk a couple of hundred metres and used that time to top up with the rest of the fluid. (400 ml pre run and 400 en-route). Then off I went. In 10 minutes I felt back to normal despite the squawking of the continuous glucose meter. This is the problem with continuous sensors. They lag a bit by about 20 minutes. They are continuous but not necessarily real-time. But I knew my meter well and liked using it. And I felt good so ignored it. In most situations like this I would just turn it off, but I was curious to see what would happen. It took about half an hour for the sensor to register the upswing due to the glucose tablets. But it all was okay to the end of the run. I even managed a small sprint at the end. I felt really good. Type 1 diabetes, 13 hour fast, 15 mile run. Job done! I picked up my medal and kept that. The goody bag I gave away. Grain and honey-based energy bar, Lucozade Sport drink, banana, popcorn, and some 'Good Stuff' 'naturally delicious' jelly sweets. I had no need of that. In fact I didn't feel like eating for another couple of hours, so I didn't.

So, what did I learn from that run? Well, the most important thing for me was that my rapid-acting insulin was now reliably cutting in at just over an hour and a half. Before I started using a ketogenic diet this was around three hours. It had been coming down gradually for several months. Insulin resistance was something I was to become obsessed with. It was eventually to drop to 40 minutes after several more months. I found that insulin resistance was not just a function of a low carbohydrate diet. Not for me anyway. It seemed to be affected

107

by the types of low carbohydrate food, my mood (including sleep), and the vagus nerve. By the end of the series of half marathons I was into a totally new field of enquiry.

A half marathon with double diabetes.

Over 20 years of injecting extra insulin to cover carbohydrate, which was unnecessary as I now know, I became insulin resistant. This was an iatrogenic illness: induced by clinicians. I had double diabetes. Type 1 and Type 2 effectively: Type 2 from the bad advice for Type 1. I was making good progress through the series of runs every month, changing things to explore possibilities. This half marathon was my home run. I was determined to prepare in the best way possible. Fast for 13 hours, as was my new routine. There were no real surprises with fasting: boring, boring beta oxidation. Beta oxidation is the metabolic process of fat burning. But, there are surprises round every corner. I got nearly to the end of that half marathon without incident, but then I turned to wave to a friend and almost fell over with dizziness. My pulse was good but fast (it is always above 160), but it was regular. What on earth was going on? My meter had given up at half way and I had no back up. Having done a basic assessment I decided it was probably nothing. I was still a bit light-headed but not confused or struggling to see, which were my usual personal warning signs of a hypo. That and extreme tiredness. I didn't have that either. There were only five minutes to go and amazingly I was on for a personal best for the year.

So in true Lemming style with only a few minutes to go I made a dash for the line. Glucose gels could wait, if they were needed at all. Having injected only a few units of basal insulin and no rapid acting insulin this would have been a slow, lazy hypo at worst. Completely different to back in the day when they would dive bomb in from nowhere. I made it to the finish without embarrassment and with nine minutes off my year's personal best. Truly remarkable! I had not achieved that time for seven years. It was something Mo Farah would likely never do. When I got round to testing about 10 minutes after the run my glucose level was 4.3 mmol/l. So starting at 6, ending at 4.3; that counted as a success.

If only...

If I knew 21 years ago what I know now I would have done so many things so differently. But I didn't. I did what I was told, and I did to others what I was taught. I believed in carb counting, DAFNE, statins. I swallowed it all, hook, line and sinker. Once you 'get it' of course, it is a light bulb moment and you wonder how it was possible to see things any other way. But that remains a minority view. I am eternally grateful to have Googled "Richard Bernstein". He changed my life, he almost certainly saved me from future problems. We will have to see. Of course, the diabetes is still there. That's going nowhere. And I feel lucky to have found fellow clinicians who also 'get' low carbing and are sharing knowledge in the hope that one day we can do better for all people with diabetes. But, I still reckon that there are plenty of clinicians who think I am completely bonkers. They will listen politely and then say something like, 'Well, good for you if it works, *for you.*' It is so infuriating. I do see genuine enthusiasm sometimes, but I guess you are only truly interested if you have the condition. All clinicians are truly interested in something. That keeps us going.

But for those of us with Type 1, it is more of a desperate search to survive. We **have** to be interested. And we need quality information. Thank goodness for the internet. Change will come from the ground up, not top down. Individuals are discovering for themselves that they can get their diabetes under control. They have discovered a tool, which enables life to be fun again. Other Lemming Test-Pilots are getting pretty slick at ketogenic dieting. It helps enormously and is life-transforming. A ketogenic-type diet is fundamental in managing Type 1 diabetes. You then learn that diet is just one part – the most important part – but you can then focus on stress management, sleep, happiness and physical activity – other great tools in the diabetes management kit.

I really hope that this has helped other diabetics, especially Type 1s, but there may be learnings for Type 2s also. I hope it has inspired anyone who is, or knows, a diabetic (that's most of us) that we can live and run without carbs or even without dietary fat – especially if we have body fat to spare. I hope it has encouraged people to take charge of their own health and at least to consider that a high carbohydrate diet really doesn't make sense for those of us who can't handle carbs.

I hope that this has reassured even Type 1 diabetics that this serious condition does not need to be one of inevitable decline.

My latest HbA1c was in the normal range and none have been in the diabetic range since I adopted a ketogenic lifestyle. Furthermore, there is no reason to expect that my HbA1c will ever go out of the normal range, as long as I stick to it. After 21 years of Type 1, even achieving an HbA1c anywhere near to normal control seems remarkable. And there will be more to gain not just by reducing carbs, but by eating real food – the most nutrient dense stuff that the planet provided for us to eat. We should be ashamed that we ever thought our factories could make anything like acceptable alternatives. The body is truly amazing if nurtured properly.

There is no 'one size fits all' model and everyone will find their own optimal diet. But, with diabetes, cutting the carbs is an essential and excellent start. It's also a huge challenge while the current dogma prevails, but it can be done and a growing number of us are doing it.

Please pass this information on. Too many people are suffering from ignorance. We are on the cusp of a paradigm change in thinking about Type 1 diabetes. The more people who know, the faster that change will happen. Please be part of the revolution.

Thank you.

Dr Ian Lake

@idlake

Chapter Six

What happened to a Swedish man diagnosed with Type 2 diabetes & a Swedish woman taking on conventional diabetes advice?

By Lars-Erik Litsfeldt

In memory of the fighter Marie Nehagen 1977-2015, founder of the Facebook Group Smart Diabetics.

My diagnosis

In the year 2000, I was diagnosed with Type 2 diabetes. This was a disease that I knew virtually nothing about, no more than that it apparently existed in two versions, one and two. When I met with a physician to go through my test results, I was given a few brochures at the end of our meeting. These were given with the best of intentions and I was most grateful. Particularly when the doctor mentioned that the pamphlets were quite costly, but I was given some thumbed copies anyway. On my way home I began to flip through the pamphlets. I read the first few pages and the news was generally positive. Diabetes was not a death sentence, but you must be sure to take care of yourself. You should change your habits and eat a healthier diet. Be careful not to eat fatty foods or drink alcohol. As I kept on reading, there were mentions of complications of the most horrible kind: blindness, amputations and heart attacks. There was a smorgasbord of issues offered to the newly fledged diabetic.

I decided to focus on the information about how to change one's diet to avoid these complications. In the morning, instead of eating bread with all sorts of good toppings, it was now porridge made of oatmeal with half a grated apple and skimmed milk.

I continued with the bread, but now I ate German whole wheat and grain bread. On the German breads, I used low-fat margarine. Low-fat margarine and low fat milk were standard in our diet in my family.

One thing that was a new experience was the low-fat cheese I used as a substitute for my regular toppings. The kindest thing I can say about this spreadable cheese version is that it tasted bad. It did not have any flavour at all. The consistency of this so-called cheese was that of hard jelly. I sought solace in the fact that it was good for me.

My heart attack

Less than a year later I had a heart attack. During a regular visit to my physician, I found out that my blood sugar levels, despite my ascetic life, had bolted to staggering numbers. I was placed on sulfonylurea medication (metformin). The kind of medication that, according to my physician, would "whip" my pancreas into shape and make sure that it would give off sufficient quantities of insulin. It sounded nasty whipping a body part, so I asked my physician if it could be good for the pancreas to be subject to such rough treatment. Perhaps it would wear out like everything else you torment, but my physician reassured me that there would be no danger to my pancreas.

When I arrived at home and started thinking about the pancreas and the harsh treatment that it would be subjected to, I felt worried despite my doctor's reassurance. Surely it could not be good for the body? I also knew that the next step in treating my diabetes would be to use syringes to dispense insulin. I never enjoyed receiving injections and the thought of giving them to myself was a most unpleasant thought. At my clinic, I had been instructed in the importance of weight loss. It was argued that my blood sugar levels would be much better if I was thinner.

My desire to lose weight was great when I felt the use of syringes coming closer. I had tried to be careful and eat the food that was recommended. Strangely enough there were no results of importance. A few kilos had disappeared but they might have been lost from taking metformin, which is the most common medication for Type 2 diabetics. I read somewhere that from the start of its use, metformin was promoted for weight loss. (Apparently, it can make people feel so nauseous and sometimes make people physically sick, so the mechanism for weight loss may not be much fun). Since I wanted to lose weight I began to frantically search the internet to see if there were any shortcuts on weight loss. After some searching, I began to see a pattern. It appeared on some pages about weight loss that you didn't have to be afraid of butter, fat or dairy products. This sounded very strange to my way of thinking and in contradiction to what I had been taught at the clinic. What would dieticians at the clinic think if they found out that I was trying the opposite to their advice? Would they faint?

Daring to eat fat

I believed that, for me as a heart patient and a diabetic, it would be a fatal blow to start eating fatty foods. On September 15, 2003, after several months of hesitation, I finally changed my diet to eat and enjoy fatty foods. My first meal was bacon and fried eggs. If, after two weeks, I felt I was dying due to my strange diet, my plan was that I would stop the experiment and return to the food that was recommended in the pamphlets and by the dieticians at the clinic. My experience on that first morning of changing my diet was amazing. I could feel that this was what the body wanted and needed all along. A day or two into my experiment, I did not dare to continue with the metformin, as I was getting shaky from the lowered blood sugar levels. The blood sugar levels had apparently improved without weight loss... I continued to enjoy my new eating habits. My appetite was huge and I ate large portions of food at both lunch and dinner, in addition to the daily breakfast of bacon and eggs. Despite my larger than average consumption of fatty foods, I lost weight. I almost felt guilty and I was at the same time still a bit concerned about my cholesterol. Surely it must have risen to astronomical numbers? I insisted on an additional test after a few weeks on my new diet. To my surprise, the results were better than the previous test. Today I would not be able to explain what good values are, but at that time I took this very seriously. I am forever grateful to the nurse who gave me the test and gave me her blessing to continue eating the new diet that had worked so well for me and my test results.

At my next appointment with the physician I explained my new diet success. She wondered what I had been doing differently since the last time since she could see that all my values and numbers had improved. I will never forget her question: "What did you say you ate for breakfast?"! Going forward I did not have to see any more of the diabetes nurses, as my physician felt that I knew at least as much as any of them about my diabetes. I could thus continue with my new eating habits.

Writing a book

Going forward a year, my friend Ulf Norrby contacted me. He had heard a headline on a radio station, about a physician specialising in diabetes who had experimented with a low carbohydrate diet with his patients. The results were surprisingly good. Ulf suggested to me "Dammit, Litsfeldt, you ought to write a book about this subject"! I was unfamiliar with how to write books but I immediately obeyed the suggestion and sat down by the computer ready to type. Since I didn't have a clue about how to write a book, I decided it probably was best to start somewhere in the middle of the story. It should probably be a chapter about fats. I started by writing "Fats" as the title and at that moment I realised that I knew virtually nothing about that either. I had to go to the bookshelf and look up the word in the encyclopedia. When I tried to understand what was written about fats, I was very close to giving up my writing project. I did not understand anything about the information given about the subject. Luckily, with the help of AltaVista on the Internet and e-mail correspondences with Dr Malcolm Kendrick and other skilled people in the field I believe I solved the question of what fat is. My understanding of the subject grew as I wrote and it was very stimulating for me.

After I was finished with the script, and following many tribulations, the book was published. It was publisher # 30 on my list that finally believed in my book and my awkward subject.

Of course, I wanted the book to be available and read by as many people as possible. I found a website that suited my requirements to spread my message about my health improvements and asked if they wanted to write about my book. I explained to them that my discovery was something that more diabetic patients should take part in and benefit from. I was surprised when I received a short e-mail in response that stated that they would not write about my book. Not that they did not want to, but they couldn't. I decided to find out more about the website origins and discovered that, like so many other sources of information about diabetes, the website was owned by a pharmaceutical company. It was my first contact with the so-called establishment, Big Pharma, concerning people with the diagnosis of diabetes.

I understand on an intellectual level that a pharmaceutical company has to make money; that is why you have a limited company. This is also why you can't spread information that harms your business. For me, it was a rude awakening and a new insight that pharmaceutical companies looked more to their profits than to the people who use the drugs they produce. You, who are reading this, might shake your head and wonder how I could be so naive. I believed that the pharmaceutical companies wanted more than to just keep their patients moderately ill for as long as possible. The sufferer shouldn't die, because then they just had lost a customer. The patient shouldn't be in full health either because financially that would be the same as if the patient were dead, or cured of whatever illness. No, a moderately ill patient, with a long life, would be the perfect customer!

It was after the release of my book that my understanding about diabetes treatment began for real. To discover a web site about diabetes treatment, which refused to take part and publish exciting information about an alternative treatment, was only the beginning. No one contacted me to learn more about my discovery.

I offered to visit my local diabetes association and give a lecture, for free. I thought a lecture about my discovery would be irresistible for an association with limited resources. Instead of the interest I expected, I found out through different channels that the President of the local diabetes association, had forwarded an email, regarding my discovery, to all diabetes associations in Sweden. In the email, she described to them that what I had discovered, had nothing to do with science and proven experience. This email was written without even talking to me about my experience. I found myself blacklisted from diabetes associations all over Sweden. It was not working out quite as I had imagined. I thought my message would raise an interest and that a lecture about this subject would be an opportunity to travel around and give talks all over Sweden. The group, which I thought would most appreciate my message, was as negative as the drug companies. That pharmaceutical companies did not appreciate me, I could understand. It was quite logical. But that my insights into diabetes were kept away from other diabetics, by their own diabetes associations... that felt strange and wrong.

Luckily there were other ways to get my message known. Thanks to the hard work of my publisher, interviews were conducted with me on the subject, by several newspapers and magazines. It was generally goodwill articles. However, the articles would always be accompanied by a disclaimer. It was as if what I had discovered and experienced was not quite true, so there had to be some kind of voice of reason to tell the reader not to be too happy about the message in the article. Fact boxes would contain statements from experts, that no matter what I said, it was familiar to all, that saturated fat was dangerous. The experts knew that there were "hundreds of thousands" of studies showing that saturated fat was the enemy of a healthy body. It was certain. There was no need for a discussion. I just couldn't find any evidence for this, however.

Annika Dahlqvist

In the autumn of 2005, a physician named Annika Dahlqvist started to blog about the impact of diet on health – a low carbohydrate diet particularly. Dahlqvist had been suffering from irritable bowel syndrome (IBS), chronic fatigue, fibromyalgia, insomnia and a cocktail of other ailments. Her daughter took part in an experiment at university, which required cutting out carbohydrates for a week and she lost weight. Curious, Dahlqvist tried the experiment for herself and found all her illnesses cleared up quickly when she cut carbohydrate and increased fat. She realised that maybe other people could be helped in a similar way and so started to spread the word via email, newsletters, blogs and the development of a nutrition programme.

Dahlqvist began to get a bit of a name for herself. The newspapers loved her because of her outspokenness. However, as other people have come to realise (Dietician Jennifer Elliott, Surgeon Dr Gary Fettke, A-rated scientist Professor Tim Noakes, as examples), dieticians don't like any advice other than their own being shared. In November 2006, two dieticians reported Dahlqvist to the Swedish National Board of Health (just as dieticians reported Elliott, Fettke and Noakes). The dieticians' complaint was that Dahlqvist's diet was not in line with that of the authorities. You bet it wasn't! That's why it was getting such great results.

The National Board appointed a special Professor to investigate whether or not a low carbohydrate diet could be considered scientific. Dahlqvist, however, was immediately impacted by the complaint – guilty until investigated, let alone verdict delivered. She lost her job at the Njurundahallen Medical centre and could no longer help her patients, in the way in which she had been doing.

The verdict was delivered in January 2008 and, tragically for the complainants, it found in favour of Dahlqvist. The National Board assessed the low carbohydrate diet as "in accordance with science and proven experience." An interesting spin on this statement is that the National Board was careful to point out that the decision related to a supervisory matter (the complaint made) and that the decision was not to be considered as dietary advice. The statement also said that the low carbohydrate diet was not sufficiently investigated in the long term and that it was important that careful follow-ups were made and recorded. It was noted that the National Board was uncomfortable with the decision, but the decision opened the doors to a more liberal view on the low carbohydrate diet in Sweden. Arguably, the dieticians would have been better off not making the complaint – they gave the low carbohydrate diet the opportunity to be 'tried' and found not guilty.

Dahlqvist was a media 'go-to' once more and she travelled extensively lecturing about her nutrition programme. She wrote several books on what was becoming known by just four letters: LCHF – Low Carb High Fat. On her blog (annikadahlqvist.com), Dahlqvist announced that she retired in May 2015 (at the age of 66). The translation of her parting statement reads as follows:

"'Food Establishment', consisting of diet professors and nutritionists, in recent years has gone to fierce counterattack against LCHF, which turns upside down their low-fat high-carbohydrate diet model that has prevailed for 40 years, supported by the food industry and pharmaceutical industry that makes money on it."

Dieticians

Dieticians and their organisation are difficult to comprehend. As with pharmaceutical companies, I wonder who they side with. Is it their dieticians' organisation and the belief systems they have been taught or is it the patient's side? The doctor that my friend Ulf Norrby told me about had good help in his study by a very interested dietician. However, this dietician's organisation found out about her interest and positive view. The pressure from her organisation made the dietician stop having a benevolent attitude to the ongoing study. One should not judge too hard. It is human to waiver when being subjected to pressure by one's own organisation. The dietician's work flipped from supporting to opposing the study, with the result that she was elected "dietician of the year" by her organisation. The doctor who ran the study, Jörgen Vesti Nielsen, was also reported to the National Board of Health by the chairman of the dietician's organisation. The National Board however, did not pursue the case.

Dieticians, as professionals, are a group that I have had a lot of interaction with. I have ended up in arguments numerous times and in all cases the dieticians withdraw. For the most part simply by stopping responding to my emails, but in one case a female dietician urged me to please not follow her blog anymore. What is difficult to understand is how they proceed with their advice to, for example, refrain from saturated fat when it turns out that they have no cause for the warnings. Instead they end the debate and continue with the warnings against saturated fat as before. In a blog posted by a dietician, it was stated: "*Thus, insulin is an essential protein needed to convert the food we eat into sugar in the blood.*" I had to read the sentence several times before it sank in that the licensed dietician was so ignorant. Insulin consequently, raises blood sugar ... right? It's scary that there are ignorant dieticians who actually think they know what they're talking about. They are given attention in the media and people believe what they say. It is equally frightening.

Saturated fat debated in Sweden

The National Food Administration (NFA) in Sweden has always said that saturated fat is dangerous. No thinking person can then understand this position, when we constantly see studies showing that it is not dangerous. How beneficial saturated fat is, I do not know. That saturated fat is not dangerous is today established beyond a reasonable doubt. Several people have, over the years, requested that the NFA should account for the scientific basis for their warnings against saturated fat. The answer that has been given is that it would be impossible because you must make an appraisal of the thousands of studies showing that saturated fat is dangerous. Apparently, this is something that only the officials of the NFA can understand and not us mere mortals.

Finally, in 2009, the NFA presented a list of 72 studies that were said to support their view that saturated fat was dangerous. In order to try to be scientific they also reported eight studies showing that saturated fat was not dangerous. Why I do not know. It ought to have rung alarm bells with the NFA when you find studies with results that contradict what you claim. In any case, one feels that it should call for a certain modesty.

When the list of the studies was published, M.D. Uffe Ravnskov along with eleven other physicians and scientists divided the cases between them. The group wanted to find out if the NFA had finally managed to scientifically show that they were right in their warnings against saturated fat. The result was a disaster for the NFA. The review resulted among other things in an article in Dagens Medicin (Today's Medicine) written by the reviewers.[1] Here are some extracts from the article:

"... Recently NFA published a list of 72 studies, which allegedly support its warnings against the saturated fat, and another list of eight studies which contradict. We have now examined this list and are dismayed. Either there is a lack of relevant basic knowledge in medical science, or else the NFA is trying to deceive us.

"... The table shows that there are two studies, which can be seen as a support; the rest can not.

"... Eleven studies are not about saturated fat.

"... A few [studies] suggest that saturated fat is healthy. Probably they have been included because the NFA's experts do not understand the meaning of their results.

"... One of the main evidences of the saturated fat innocence; Ronald Krauss discovered that the strongest risk marker among the lipids is a high concentration of small, dense LDL particles, and that their number increases when reducing the intake of saturated fat and thereby increases the amount of carbohydrates, and vice versa. The implication of this discovery has apparently not been understood by the NFA, because two such studies have been perceived as support for dietary advice.

"... The administration's list of eight studies that are said to speak against dietary advice (I-VIII) gives a touch of scientific openness, but is at least incomplete. For example, it has ignored the many studies that have shown that people who revel in saturated fat do not have higher cholesterol or are more atherosclerotic than others. And where are the numerous studies that have shown that the infarct and

stroke patients have not eaten more saturated fat than others? ... There are at least 30 more, including six that have shown that stroke patients are eating less saturated fat than others.

"... The public should be informed that the warnings against the saturated fat lacks all credibility. It is time for the responsible people in power to decide that the NFA should immediately stop providing dietary advice to the public and leave the matter to the people with clinical experience and adequate scientific training."

Perhaps the most serious criticism still came from the newspaper's editor Per Gunnar Holmgren. It was namely an attempt at a debate between the NFA and the group of reviewers but it fizzled out when the NFA withdrew. The NFA argued among other things that the reviewers probably did not understand the meaning of the studies because they were not sorted correctly. A strange argument since the review team consisted of plenty of people with a scientific background. Among them was, notably among others, the former secretary of the Medical Research Council, Tore Scherstén. He who at the time was the NFA's spokesman was not even a Ph.D. So wrote Holmgren:

"Can the NFA not answer?

"... Without taking a position in the noisy discussion of dietary recommendations, I can state that the critical writers set forward a maximum of legitimate questions ...

"...I can also see that the NFA in its response, entirely avoided giving specific answers to questions that authority must be able to answer. We are still awaiting an answer – this time, a real response."

The NFA responded twice on the review group's criticism, but it managed to answer without touching what the criticism was concerned. They even managed to avoid mentioning the term "saturated fat". Holmgren wrote:

"NFA's strategy seems incomprehensible. Why doesn't the NFA give more effort to give their critics a sustainable response? How is it credible to argue that the dietary advice is based on "sound scientific facts" and then not be able to report or discuss these scientific works."

It is reasonable to believe that the NFA after this heavy defeat would consider changing its position or at least launch an investigation as to whether you need to revise the dietary advice to the population. However, the warnings continue today. The fact that NFA stated that the dietary advice is based on broad scientific principles, even after this debacle, is actually ridiculous and that is sad.

In 2008, the work to develop a new dietary guideline for people suffering from diabetes began. A group of experts drew up proposals for these suggested guidelines. As it turned out, two of the members of the group were too closely involved with the business community and particularly in the food industry. It was the newly appointed head of the National Board of Health who took the decision to remove them. Nils Georg Asp and Bengt Vessby had, among others, co-operated with the Swedish Nutrition Foundation, a lobbying organisation funded by 40 food companies. They had previously assisted in developing a brochure for diabetics and heart patients called "Good food for you," a brochure that would inform the patients of what was advisable to eat. This was one of the pamphlets I received from the hospital when I was first diagnosed with my diabetes. The idea was to simplify for the patients and so therefore there were examples of what you could eat in a day. Please remember that this menu was written for those who can't properly process sugar and starch:

For breakfast, it was suggested to eat oatmeal with a grated apple and skim milk. To this one could add bread with toppings. Since breakfast consisted mostly of simple carbohydrates, a snack would be needed a couple of hours later. The snack suggestion was a sugared bun and coffee. For lunch, one option was to eat vegetables, macaroni, fried lean sausage and a piece of bread. Most people who ate anything like this meal, would know that satiety does not continue and therefore it was also required to have a snack in the afternoon as well. A fruit salad was suggested for the afternoon snack. It should be mentioned that a banana contains as much sugar and starch as the amount of glucose in 12 sugar cubes. Dinner could be salad, rice, fish in foil, a sandwich, a glass of beer, vegetables and fruit. The menu proposal ended with a glass of skim milk and a sandwich as an evening snack. In another brochure for diabetics there were hints as how to treat a person who fell into an insulin induced coma – this would be a person who has taken too much insulin. In these cases, one could, according to this brochure, try to give the person (who is ill) five glucose tablets or a glass of milk. As you may gather, this snack contains enough sugar to bring back a half-dead person to life. An eye-opener as to whether the brochure on food for diabetics is good for diabetics or for the food producers.

Those who helped to produce this brochure were thus stumbling close to being involved in developing modern dietary advice for diabetics. I give a thought of gratitude to the Head of the National Board who took them away. So, what happened to the now delayed dietary advice? One can sum it up in what is reported in the Swedish Diabetes Association's brochure "*Let yourself be inspired.*" Essentially, those tasked with coming up with the optimal dietary advice for diabetics decided upon four diets – not one:

- Traditional diabetic diet;

- Diabetic diet with low Glycaemic Index (GI);

- Moderate carbohydrate diet;

- Mediterranean Diet.

The traditional diabetic diet is basically about eating low fat products (which are thus high carb). "Don't eat too much" is usually part of this advice (ignoring how hungry you get). Diabetic diet plus low GI adds a "choose lower GI foods" condition to the already low fat high carb diet. Moderate carb is all of this, but worry about the carbs less. The Mediterranean Diet is the most misunderstood of all. Anyone who has been to the region knows that the real Mediterranean Diet is all about eating animals and white things. The animals include everything from snails to horse with cheese and cream welcome. The white things are refined, rather than whole, grains – French bread sticks, Panini, pasta, pizza, risotto rice etc. The real Mediterranean Diet, minus white things, is actually therefore a good starting place for diabetes. It can be naturally low carb high fat (LCHF) – where you should not be afraid of consuming natural fats and stay away from white products and carbohydrates.

It is strange that two such diametrical opposites – LFHC and LCHF – can be accommodated in the same dietary advice. One of the diets ought to reasonably be better than the other, and then the other diet wouldn't be there? I am aware that we are all a little different and that we can feel good from the different composition of nutrients. From experience, I know that many diabetics who stuck to the recommended diet experience a great health improvement when they changed over to the LCHF diet. I tried a little unscientific test by eating according to the brochure "*Good food for all*" during a few days. A few days earlier I had tested my blood sugar, just a couple of hours after breakfast and the number was around 6, it oscillated between 5.5 and 7. When I tested my blood sugar during my experiments with oatmeal porridge and accessories, instead, the blood sugar was now well over 12. A blood sugar that is obviously harmful.

So, at this point a low carbohydrate diet, however moderate, is a recommended diet for diabetics in Sweden. A lot has happened since Annika Dahlqvist was reported by the two dieticians. No one could have imagined how these two dieticians sped up the process of getting a low carbohydrate diet approved as an alternative diet for diabetics. Instant karma. And why not a statue?

Before concluding this chapter, I would like to go back in time to show the bizarre detour the councils have taken.

The aversion to allowing diabetics to eat fat and especially saturated fat, is due to the cholesterol hypothesis. It is based on the theory that a high level of cholesterol in the blood causes heart disease. Diabetics are very likely to have heart attacks so what could be better than to warn diabetics from eating fat? Increasing protein intake is not good for a diabetic, since glucose can be formed by protein and thus raise blood sugar. The remaining nutrients are alcohol and carbohydrates. When insulin's role was discovered, it was advised to stay away from non blood sugar raising fats and instead eat carbohydrates – the nutrient that raises blood sugar the most. Blood sugar could of course be lowered with insulin so what was the problem? Today we know that it is sugar that is the major culprit when it comes to heart disease.

Before the hyperglycemic dietary advice was developed, diabetics were recommended to eat as many fatty foods as possible. In the 1910s, Professor Karl Petrén, a successful diabetic specialist in Sweden, understood that carbohydrates made diabetics worse and instead recommended fatty food. Before him starvation was a popular method to keep the blood sugar levels to a minimum. He was also ahead of his time in recommending caution about protein, which can be converted to glucose. Potatoes was something he forbade, while he allowed 100 grams of bread per day. Petrén knew of course that the bread was very bad for a diabetic but he also knew that bread was almost impossible to stop eating. We know today that bread contains opioids. Instead of completely banning bread, he therefore allowed a limited amount. He knew that a total ban of bread would only make his patients ignore the advice completely. Better to lower the level of ambition and instead hope that bread intake would be quite small.

In Petrén's book from 1926,[2] *"On the treatment of diabetes (also with insulin)"* the author presented the conclusion that:

" diabetes is a metabolic disturbance, characterized by the inability of the body to utilize sugar at a normal rate...only in this way can it be successfully treated, and that is by the choice of a proper diet, and by adhering to certain limitations regarding the diet. In this way, improvement can be achieved. By improvement I mean that the relevant symptoms of the disease disappear."

These are strong words, indeed. Further down, Petrén states that

"improvements can, however, also be then observed in that the weakness of the pancreas, that is, reduction of its internal secretion to the blood (production of insulin), is partially reversed."

This would indicate that diabetes can be reversed. This is in stark contrast to what is stated in contemporary books about diabetes, which imply that a diabetic must follow the so-called natural course of events and succumb to a disease that continually and increasingly destroys their health. In the past, they left the door open for improvement. This sounds exciting, so we continue:

"Seemingly, any of these types of improvement can only be achieved by subjecting oneself to certain restrictions in the diet, and the outlook for persistent improvement can only be achieved by a single means, mainly that the diabetes sufferer shall forever continue to subject himself to such restrictions regarding the diet, as in the given case are necessary. It is thusly not a simple cure, but a question of changing lifestyle."

In those days, diet was the keystone of diabetes treatment. Petrén also contemplated the question of daily calorie intake:

"If the required quantity of foodstuff is consumed, the person in question will be of stable body weight. If a larger quantity is consumed, one will under certain circumstances increase the body weight, which, however, is by no means certain; it is well-known that certain persons, who are persistently lean, may profess to a ravenous appetite. If, on the contrary, less than the required amount of foodstuff is consumed, the inevitable result is a decrease in weight."

This is an interesting paragraph. Petrén concludes that it is not at all certain that eating a lot will result in weight gain.

Fat was by then, before the insulin treatment, the nutrient that should keep the diabetics alive as long as possible. After the discovery of insulin, diabetics didn't need to be so careful about trying to keep the blood sugar level down naturally. Many decades have passed and the knowledge of a natural way to control blood sugar levels has largely been forgotten. However, the last few years has rejuvenated interest and the escalating incidence of diabetes has acquired a new urgency. Hopefully we'll not have to see fat-rich dietary advice once again be overlooked. Major economic interests of course want the natural method of control of blood sugar to be forgotten or to appear dangerous. Now it's up to you and me to constantly remind the public about these fatty diets.

Lars-Erik Litsfeldt

Diabetes, No thanks! Little Moon Publishing 2011

Chapter Seven

What can a man do when diagnosed with Type 2 Diabetes? (Fixing Dad)

by Jen Whitington

Once upon a time...

I remember hearing a story when I was little called 'The King and the Mirror of Truth'. In the story an old king woke up one day and looked in the mirror. He was startled and horrified by the reflection staring back at him. In that stark moment he was forced to face the reality of what he had become: a bloated, jowly, sallow-skinned old man. The light of youth that had once shone in his eyes had long been extinguished leaving only the hollow and indifferent gaze that now confronted him.

He was distraught and called his various courtiers to tell him that the mirror had lied. Cautiously and tactfully they each told him that this was, in truth who he had become and quietly left the room. Each of them, that is, except for the jester. Left alone with the crumpled king he smiled and asked him if he doubted the mirror. 'Yes,' he said, 'I have never looked so terrible in all my life. Has life marked me so strikingly to have taken my youth, my vigour, my soul?'

The jester smiled, 'There is only one way to find out sire but it is a long and arduous quest. If you want the honest answer to that question you must find 'The Mirror of Truth'.

The king brightened, 'I will do anything to find it if it can show me that there is anything left of the man I once was,' he said. The jester smiled and told him he must prepare and pack for a long journey as they must leave immediately.

In the story the king left with the jester and they spent many exhausting and gruelling months travelling across the kingdom together. Despite the trials and challenges they laughed and joked

127

heartily together and with the people they met along the way. Away from the comforts and confines of the palace the king began to look on his life and his kingdom very differently.

Finally, after months of traveling, they came across a ruined castle and inside an old dilapidated hall was a mirror. The king looked on eagerly as the jester glanced into it and told him that this was indeed the mirror that they had been looking for. With great trepidation the king stepped up to the mirror. There, staring back at him, was a strong, lean man with a wizened face and the fire of purpose in his eyes.

'This is The Mirror of Truth, sire and this is your true self,' said the jester. 'You will only ever see who you really are in a reflection outside the walls that limit you. It is only by looking outside those walls that you will see everything that you are. Never lose sight of this reflection, your majesty. It is this that will guide you and shape who you have yet to become.' He paused and watched the king who stood intently memorising his reflection. The same tired old man that had left the palace was now glowing with the realisation of what it is to be alive. He smiled, 'Shall we return home, sire?'

'This kingdom is my home jester,' smiled the king. 'Each one of the once strangers, now friends, is my family. I am lucky to have met them all and now it is my duty to unite them together. Every one of them must complete a journey of their own but they will only truly enjoy it with the warmth of honest companionship. Should I live to be a hundred, I will never be able to thank you enough.'

The Whitington Family

I was about eight years old when I heard this story and it had always stuck with me somewhere at the very back of my mind. The day it came back in full colour was quite unexpected – on so many levels. It was the day I watched my glowing and athletic father in law, Geoff, cross the finish line of a supremely challenging 100 mile cycle event in London in August 2014.

Unexpected because only ten months before Geoff had been facing the very real threat of a diabetic amputation. He had been diagnosed with Type 2 diabetes nine years previously but he hadn't been in good health for decades. He had been overweight and overly stressed for most of his adult life. Erratic and harsh working hours, night shifts, financial strain and a kind of smash and grab approach to his diet and health was catching up with him at a galloping pace. For the most part, Geoff was indifferent. At 62 he had to accept that he was getting older and with that came the resignation that ill health seemed to be an inseparable part of the ageing process. As far as Geoff was concerned his medication would fend off the worst of the problems. At the same time though, he knew it wasn't. His doctor had upped his metformin to four a day with gliclazide thrown into the mix. The next step was injecting insulin.

The quizzical engineer side of him wondered why, if the pills were doing their job, did he keep having to take more of them? And why were they not preventing these other complications from cropping up? His left foot was now deformed by the onset of Charcot foot (a result of diabetic neuropathy that had caused the arch in the foot to collapse entirely) making walking extremely painful and impossible without his air boot. The toes on his right foot were worryingly covered with black diabetic ulcers that needed repeated attention but, despite that, they wouldn't go away. How was he to be expected to follow the half hearted prescription of 'diet and exercise' if he was essentially immobile and when all movement threatened to complicate his foot problems still further? He'd really sharpened his resolve on the diet front too: nothing focuses the mind, or turns the stomach, quite like the threat of amputation. But even his recommended diet wasn't working. If anything it seemed to be making him heavier and even more tired.

Geoff began to accept ongoing and accelerating deterioration. His condition, according to his original GP was 'lifelong and manageable' – hardly the kind of inspiring language needed to motivate a patient to make the kind of diet and lifestyle changes that could alleviate the misery. Life long and manageable suggests 'permanent and worsening' so why make life still more unpleasant with the kind of self-recriminations that followed every slip off the wagon? Perhaps he'd be better off not boarding the wagon than feeling the sharp sting of failure every time he fell off it?

Geoff knew there were certain actions he definitely needed to take: he snapped up every night shift and bit of overtime he could in an attempt to leave his finances in a better state when the inevitable happened. He was ill, exhausted and broken. To his mind, he was on borrowed time.

His family looked on and felt helpless. Lecturing him had never worked – Geoff is a proud and stubborn man. In his own words 'I know what I need to be doing but I'm not going to be doing it, all right?' Frustration, anger, blame and guilt made frequent appearances in these desperate conversations to get Geoff to ditch his destructive habits – but they had no effect. It was with the talk of amputation that his two sons, Anthony and Ian, sat down together and decided they weren't ready to lose their dad, even one piece at a time. Their dad was falling apart and they needed a plan to fix him.

Step 1: Get the facts

Googling a health condition is a terrifying process but that was the only place his sons could think to start. The language, case studies, prognosis (both on an individual and population level) and future sufferer projections are bleak and depressing. And even worse this disease, and its complications, are everywhere. It was no wonder that both Geoff and his original GP were as numb to this diagnosis as Geoff's feet were to a pair of nail scissors. The magnitude of the task ahead of his sons started to hit them both.

They knew Geoff's diet needed to change and that he urgently needed to lose weight to alleviate the strain on his feet. They knew that they needed to do what they could to get his blood glucose stable. They also knew that the word 'moderation' in terms of their dad's old culinary favourites was very much a subjective one. At the height of his excesses (and coincidentally, the lowest ebb in his mental health) Geoff had been known to make 3-7 trips to a drive-thru in a day. In Geoff's lenient, loop-hole seeking interpretation of 'moderation', one trip a day would be positively abstemious. Nonetheless, avoiding those places entirely would be better. A particular point of frustration for the boys was that their dad knew this but still he kept doing it. Why? Habit? Cost efficiency (more food for his money and endless budget deals)? Familiarity? Meaning? Identity? Comfort? Welcome escape from the bland, low calorie foods he was told to consume? They started to realise that there was a great deal more to the lifestyle that had quite literally shaped their dad than just grabbing a meal.

Step 2: Get the trust

They knew that before they could even begin to tackle his diet, they needed to somehow jemmy their way into his mind and decided to accomplish this on an uncomfortable and emotionally turbulent road trip to Spain. The love and closeness between these three is compelling to watch. After some painful and tearful conversations about why their dad's health was so important to them, why it should be a priority to him too, and the harsh reality that neither of them were in a position to care for him physically or financially should the complications get worse (and so showing him that his health is intrinsically their business) they also reminded him of all the positive things he had to live for, which he was so apt to forget as he'd become more accustomed at looking at the bleak picture ahead of him. They told him they'd get the weight off him and that he would have more energy. They assured him that it didn't have to be an uncomfortable process about denial and will power. And above all they assured him that they would be right there with him through all of it.

Slowly they were able to break down most of the self imposed barriers that Geoff had to taking charge of his own health but this was an ongoing process. Through the family's later work with hundreds of other Type 2 diabetics they found a common and recurring theme that they saw in these early days with Geoff. At the start of this process there was a significant mental hurdle that Anthony and Ian had to get over and it is one we have seen too often since. Geoff, like so many Type 2 diabetics had a shameful, and often buried, sense that he had done this to himself. He had overeaten, over indulged, never taken any formal exercise (although his career had been hugely physically active, his 'retirement' job as a night-time security guard was sedentary but he wasn't slim in either role). As far as he was concerned he'd brought this upon himself. He didn't deserve sympathy or help. It was his fault and beating this disease – if that was even an option – would be like cheating. Geoff believed in fair consequences and this was the justice he should have expected all along.

His sons, on the other hand, took it as a challenge and refused to let it beat them. After some serious digging they were able to show their dad that he wasn't to blame – certainly not as much as he thought. He'd spent years doing his best to follow mainstream, conventional dietary guidelines that his particular body couldn't cope with so there was no way it would be able to cope with indulgences or excesses beyond that. That meant that not only did he *deserve* to be healthy but that there was every chance he could be. They also knew they had to get their dad feeling differently, and quickly, if they stood any chance of getting his buy-in.

On their road trip to Spain, Anthony and Ian had to start from scratch. They had to teach their dad how to cook anything at all and then how to cook some new ingredients that he had never used before. These mostly fell into the bracket of being 'green' or having come 'out of the sea'. Geoff's usual food consumption fell into a bracket that you could label 'beige'. He was no stranger to dietary regimes and this was just another one as far as he was concerned. His expectations weren't high and, if his sons were going to continue to enforce that he eat 'weird' stuff just as some kind of entertaining sport for their own purposes, then he would immediately abandon it. All three of them knew too well that Geoff was never going to just abandon it though. He was far too stubborn for that and that particular character trait was going to need to be fully maximised if they were to use it to their advantage.

Step 3: Get the grub

Back in 2013 when this all began for the family, the idea of a diet low in carbohydrates to treat and manage Type 2 diabetes was not so clearly publicised as it is now. Geoff's oldest son, Anthony, was diagnosed pre diabetic at this time too. As his wife I found this very difficult to understand. Because of our large family I had always made our meals from scratch as I found it to be more economical so I knew there couldn't be any added nasties in there causing some kind of metabolic mayhem. Besides, at the time he was fit and well. He was frequently running half marathons, competing in national Kung Fu tournaments and had a healthy BMI of 25. He rarely drank alcohol either. It wasn't as though he was overweight or a stereotypical case. He was told that he most likely had a genetic predisposition to the condition, which is probably true but it doesn't make it acceptable to confused loved ones and we knew too well where persistently raised blood glucose ended up so we also knew we had to sort that too.

Anthony's pre diabetes was perhaps where we as a family learned the most. It wasn't until we completely grasped the concept of 'No GPS' (grains, potatoes and sugar) that we started to see his HbA1c readings normalise and so realised that, despite Geoff being a long way down the diabetic road, we could follow the same principles with him. Geoff's packets of beige took a while to banish entirely but when he watched how they spiked blood glucose readings when he checked them, he could make immediate sense for himself of the damage those foods were doing to him. His 'turning a blind eye' became the scrutinising gaze of intrigue as he tracked and followed his body's response to food until food preparation and meal times became far more intuitive and enjoyable as a result. Just as his sons had promised, it wasn't so tough either. He replaced the lazy beige with meat, fish, eggs, full fat dairy products and lots of green veg.

Everything was not only tastier and more varied, it was also more interesting and, best of all, Geoff started to feel his energy levels rise again. It was at this point that his sons convinced him to do the odd short ride on his bike. His bike had been a whole family birthday present a few years before. It had a specially adapted frame to support his weight. Geoff had only used it once in that time to go and pick up some kebabs. His conclusion was that it was unfit for this purpose as cycling with carrier bags on the handlebars was awkward and probably dangerous so the bike was stowed away in the furthest, darkest, most inaccessible recesses of his garage to ensure that he didn't feel tempted to do another takeaway run on it in the future. Besides that, Geoff had an inbuilt fear of exercising alone. This became obvious when he briefed both his sons in CPR. They were going to have to exercise together if Geoff was going to gain confidence and start to feel safe.

So, what can a man do? Or achieve, more like...

In the seven months that followed his sons' intervention, Geoff went from nearly 20 stone (127 kg) to just under 13 stone (82 kg). His sons caught the whole journey in their BBC documentary '*Fixing Dad*' and worked hard to get the story out to as many other sufferers as they could in the hope of fixing them too. They became rather frustrated by the media focus on the before and after photos of their dad. They knew that these were the pictures that everyone understood but for them, the before and after photos they preferred were those from the MRI scanner. Those showed the fat that Geoff had stripped out of his liver and pancreas that led to the magical confirmation from Professor Roy Taylor (Head of Metabolic Medicine at Newcastle University) that their dad's Type 2 diabetes was 'resolved'.

But there were so many things that none of those photos could ever show. Geoff had found his excitement for life again. He'd rediscovered the depth of love felt for him across his family. He'd found out that he seriously loved cycling and that it was ideal for him as it didn't drive too much weight through his feet. Those ailing feet that had anchored him to his armchair just a few months ago, now powered him through hundreds of miles of the British countryside and continue to today, three years later, as he prepares for this summer's hundred miler. He still loves a pub lunch but doesn't think twice about asking if they can replace the chips with greens and he'll happily cycle miles to get to it. He vehemently says that he could never go back to the way he was. He still has the legacy of years of diabetes to deal with: specially adapted shoes, frequent checks with the podiatrist, spot checks of his blood glucose readings which, thankfully, continue to be well within normal range. But, to his great delight, he is no longer ruled by pills. Under supervision he has been off all his diabetes medications all this time, and several other medications too.

Three years may have passed since Geoff and his sons started their journey but Geoff frequently says he feels better than he has in decades. The family continue to spread their experiences across the world believing that the language and messages around Type 2 diabetes can be changed to one of hope and not helplessness. Geoff remains convinced that if a 'stubborn old git' like him can do it, anyone can and the emails that come in from people saying that they have done just that after watching the documentary, give him more pleasure than we could have imagined. With each one of these heartfelt and deeply personal stories the truth that Type 2 diabetes can be both prevented and halted clamours louder than ever.

We believed that it was going to take a massive lifestyle overhaul to see any change in Geoff's condition. We were wrong. All it took was for a few small and consistent changes to start adding up. But just as importantly it was the love and support that made it worthwhile.

Geoff, Anthony and Ian all look back and call it the best few years of their lives and, yes, the reflection that now looks back from the mirror shows a happy, healthy and purposeful man who continues to enjoy the most rewarding of adventures: a new lease of life.

You can read the full story and watch the film at www.fixingdad.com

Jen Whitington

@FixingDad
fixingdad.com
Fixing Dad: How to save someone you love, Short Books 2016

Case Study: Nigel

In six months following diagnosis, Nigel Fowler went from literally being at death's door, to being "fitter than he had been since a teenager"; despite the medical profession telling him he was "too well too soon"!

I am a 47-year old property manager in Lancashire. I share my home with my stepdaughter and five dogs. I am also a trustee of a small charity which cares for wild birds in distress, and help manage the charity's collection of wildlife reserves.

Life for me has presented some challenges along the way; I was very ill for the first 12 months of my life, which sadly claimed the life of my twin brother despite the hospital's best efforts.

I was a pretty fit and active youngster and enjoyed cross-country running at school, and was an avid member of Cubs, Scouts, and Venture Scouts, attaining both Chief Scouts Award and Queen's Scout Award along the way.

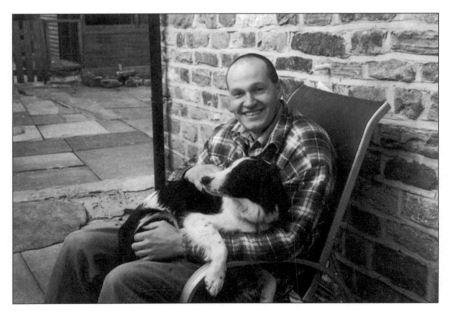

My first major health scare was in 1988. I had become very lethargic, to the point of exhaustion. A gland that had risen – but deemed harmless – in the previous year, was now a cancerous lump that had spread to 95% of my thyroid.

What followed was three major operations, nearly six months off work, and medication for life – but hey, I was still here!

Fast forward to 2011, and a change in job meant that the 18-hour days that I had been used to for 15 years disappeared. I soon put on a 'bit of a middle' – spare tyre if you like, but didn't carry any weight elsewhere.

At my heaviest I was 16 st 2 lbs, which at 6'3" was not too bad.

Come June 2014, I noticed that I was drinking quite a lot of water, and food didn't taste as sweet any more (I put this down to the chocolate and cake manufacturers altering their recipes). I also developed what I thought was a persistent urinary tract infection (UTI).

I was also having sleepless nights, leaving me with a fuzzy head and unclear sight the following day.

I put the whole thing down to a particularly stressful year with my new employer.

But the symptoms wouldn't go away and by the time I booked a GP's appointment in mid-November, I had lost two stone in weight, was going to the toilet several times a night, and my UTI was incredibly painful.

My GP took a fasting blood glucose test, and I expected the results a few days later. He actually called within 24 hours with an order: get to hospital urgently!

Mine were the highest readings they had ever seen!

I was at the local diabetic clinic within the hour. A further hour later, and I was on the insulin which would prove to be life-saving. My HbA1c at diagnosis was 101 mmol/mol.

It may seem strange, but I was incredibly grateful to be diagnosed diabetic. I had felt so ill, that I feared it was cancer again. I just didn't think I would have been strong enough this time to fight it.

As health professionals debated which type of diabetes I had, it really didn't matter to me. Yes, I was diabetic, but it wasn't cancer. I knew that I would beat this myself.

I spent the following weeks taking six daily injections and measuring my bloods. Although my levels were coming down, they were prone to huge swings and left me feeling terrible.

I was encouraged to continue on my regular diet, as my insulin rates had been calculated to a 'usual' diet. This meant lots of cake, bread, and cereal, whether I felt like them or not.

I was also told off by my Diabetes Specialist Nurse for dropping my HbA1c too quickly; from 101 to 51 in 6 months was 'too quick' and risked a relapse; the first time I have been told off for being too well!

I started researching the benefits of a LCHF lifestyle, and it all made sense. The moment I started following it, I knew it was right. WOW – what a difference.

Many people had written about huge weight losses, but it immediately calmed the yo-yo effect on my blood sugars.

I had signed up for a DAFNE (Dose Adjustment For Normal Eating) course, and they encouraged me to go back on my old diet. All I had to do was match those carbs with insulin, but that sent my blood sugars yo-yoing.

I was back to LCHF within a week, and haven't looked back.

(I will say that I am VERY grateful to the DAFNE course, as it was hugely useful in many other ways; especially in giving me the freedom to live my life as unhindered as possible.)

With my blood glucose steadying out and lowering, I gradually reduced, and then stopped, my daily insulin injections.

And how has this affected my life? Well, I really feel like a new man.

I am fitter, healthier, can run up a hill I have only been able to walk up, and even have shed some of those surplus pounds.

Friends and family are so impressed with my improved health, that they are looking into the benefits of an LCHF lifestyle – whether they are diabetic or not. I'm so glad to say that my daughter has taken the leap.

For anyone who has just been diagnosed with diabetes, I know it will be a shock, but you CAN beat it.

The key really is to reduce those high sugars as soon as you can. If you adopt a low-carb lifestyle, you won't need such invasive medication, and your health as a whole will improve. I would like to take the opportunity to thank Dr David Unwin for his support and willingness to help me along my diabetic journey, in particular with regard to LCHF.

Don't worry about your cravings for carbs: they disappear remarkably quickly, as there is no need to snack as you are always feeling full between meals.

(In fact, eating carbs really doesn't fill you up for long at all – you just end up craving more food; it's no wonder I put on so much weight).

As time goes on you learn how different foods are used by your body, and you can make some very interesting dishes.

Being told I was diabetic gave me a new zest for life – this was an illness I could do something about. A motto of mine is "Knowledge is best when shared" and I now enjoy sharing my experience with others.

In fact, you'll regularly find me chatting on the global forum for diabetes (www.diabetes.co.uk), and I'd be happy to share thoughts and ideas with you there.

Practitioners

Chapter Eight

How did a LFHC dietitian become LCHF?

by Dr Caryn Zinn, Ph.D

"Why do we advise people with diabetes to eat mostly carbohydrate foods, the very nutrient that they can't easily tolerate?"

This head-scratching question – put to me by a colleague, almost 5 years ago now – was one of the first to kick off my journey into what I can only describe as my nutrition awakening. As a dietitian, with almost 20 years of loyalty to the trusty high carb low fat nutrition mantra, my 180 degree turn in philosophies came as much of a surprise to me as it did to anyone else. What follows is an insight into my journey, my work now as an "LCHF dietitian", success stories in my consulting clinic, and some interesting stories of "backlash" in Southern hemisphere Down Under.

That "Damascus" moment

Born and bred in Cape Town, South Africa I studied a physiology degree and a dietetics degree; an emigration to New Zealand saw me studying Masters and Ph.D degrees and working in public health (initially), and then in academia and private practice. Essentially, that means I went through 11 years of study of nutrition-related qualifications, four graduation ceremonies, and almost 20 years of work without ever thinking to ask a single question about how our nutrition guidelines came to be, and simply accepting that that is just how it was. It embarrasses me now to think about this, perhaps it was a combination of the power of dogma and the fact that my experience of undergraduate student life was to "get taught" rather than to "figure out". My turn to enquire began when I started post-grad study, but by that stage, dogma had made sure that, whatever my research question, it was set firmly in the one-tracked dimension of high carb, low fat nutrition.

I currently work as an academic at AUT (Auckland University of Technology) in New Zealand, in a research unit called The Human Potential Centre, and as a private practice dietitian. I have always maintained my private practice work, as I find it keeps me grounded in reality (and busy!). It was about 5 years ago when my nutrition world as I knew it came crashing down. Now if you know anything about academia and academics you will know that there are some "interesting" personality types in this setting. My colleague, Professor of Public Health, Grant Schofield is one of those interesting personalities, and I mean this in the most flattering possible way. Being full of passion for his specialist area, physical activity and wellness, he frequently flies into the office with an exciting new, often "out there", health concept or research idea, rants about it for a few weeks before he's onto the next thing. Naturally, when he flew into the office one day ranting about low carb, high fat diets and the problems with our current nutrition guidelines, I figured it was my job (because I'm the dietitian) to put him straight. So, I spouted off what I had been taught, which is what I taught my students, and what I advised my clients: "Carbohydrate is the dominant energy source for the body; the brain can only use carbohydrate as fuel; you need carbohydrate for B vitamins and fibre; low carbohydrate diets are dangerous; fat is calorie dense and too much of it is unhealthy and will prevent you from losing weight; saturated fat gives you heart disease; ketosis is a dangerous state for the body to be in..." and so it continued.

Unfortunately (or looking back, fortunately) for me, that didn't keep Grant quiet – not a lot does when it's not physiologically and biochemically sound (funny that!). His response was this: "But the body runs perfectly well on fat as a fuel, surely that's obvious, otherwise we wouldn't have survived as a species; the brain can use ketones as a fuel source; surely you can get B vitamins and fibre from other foods? Low carb diets are equally as good for weight loss as low fat diets and better for improving health conditions. And actually, saturated fat does not give you heart disease according to the research I've read".

When he came back with all this, I went from being mildly annoyed to outraged. He had obviously been reading erroneous material and bad science, and what's more, nutrition was not his area of expertise and I figured that he should just stick to what he's qualified to do i.e., physical activity research. I honestly thought he was just being "davfa" – a beautiful word of Yiddish origin, used often in my family, which means 'just to annoy, just to be contrary'.

How naive was I at that point in time?

But then we entered into a discussion about insulin resistance and diabetes and he asked why we (as in dieticians and other health professionals) manage Type 2 diabetes, a condition characterised by insulin resistance (i.e., a pseudo carbohydrate-intolerance) with a carbohydrate-dominant diet? That, considering carbohydrate is not even an essential nutrient and can be made by the body from other substrates (another concept I had never really considered in this context).

Suddenly, what I had always taught and practised, didn't seem logical to me. I had never actually thought about these issues, but naturally, believed that there must be a good reason for carbohydrates being as important as they're made out to be in mainstream nutrition guidance systems and clinical practice. After all, our national guidelines are referred to as "best practice". I figured the only thing to do was to go away and dig up the evidence that justified these concepts, and while I was at it, the evidence supporting our daily requirements of 6-11 serves of grains, 2 serves of fruit, 3 serves of vegetables, 2 serves of low fat dairy and 1 serve of meat. That would set the record straight, and force Grant to move on to his next great idea... in the area of physical activity, that is.

The search began...

Being an academic, you soon learn what constitutes good, ok, and bad evidence. You become a nit-picker and at times, you find yourself playing devil's advocate, but you need to have this attention to detail to make sure the research is up to scratch. After all, research informs practice and if it's wrong, then we're in trouble. Hhhmm you only have to look at the trajectory of our health statistics, particularly diabetes, to get a feel of just how wrong we've been.

145

So, taking the hierarchies of evidence into consideration, what we know is that people's opinions and case studies (i.e., n=1 studies) are considered the lowest level of evidence (academically speaking, that is), randomised controlled trials (RCTs) and analyses of these (meta-analyses) are considered the highest and most robust levels of evidence, while observational studies are somewhere in the middle.[1] The main reason for this is because RCTs, or intervention trials, if conducted well and analysed properly, can show a cause-and-effect relationship. Observational studies, irrespective of how long they are and how many people they include can only show a correlation or association-type relationship. Don't get me wrong, associations are important, especially strong ones, but once established, they need further testing in RCTs to confirm cause-and-effect.

It will come as no surprise to you, the reader, that I didn't bring a lot to the table in terms of *robust* evidence.

- There was plenty of observational literature showing benefits of wholegrains for health. But was the benefit coming from the wholegrain itself or from its vitamin or mineral components? – which incidentally can be found in other (unprocessed) foods.

- There was plenty of literature supporting high carb, low fat diets in relation to health and disease, but again these were largely observational studies, many filled with methodological holes and assumptions about causal factors.

- There was RCT-based literature showing that the high carb, low fat diet trumps the standard American diet for weight loss and health outcomes, but then most diets would if you look at the sorry state of the comparison diet in these studies.

But, evidence justifying macronutrient distribution thresholds, and food group serving sizes simply didn't exist at the hierarchical level at which I was seeking. In fact all I could find was that these were developed merely as a way to more easily meet the vitamin and mineral thresholds, as specified in the NRVs (nutrient reference values), or DRIs (dietary reference intakes, originally known as the RDAs, Recommended Dietary Allowances). As for these thresholds, they were set from available evidence at the time i.e., in the 1940s, which included nutrient intake data observed in apparently normal, healthy people, epidemiological observations of populations where nutrient deficiencies were corrected by dietary improvement, and animal study extrapolations. Ok, scientists made do with what they had at the time, and they have been updated over the years, but again the precise nature of the system is far from perfect.

Suffice to say, I was beginning to see some holes in this wider nutrition story.

This literature scrutiny only sparked my interest to go further down the murky rabbit warren on other areas of the debate, in particular the saturated fat / heart disease issue and the science surrounding sugar, carbs, insulin, and low carb, high fat diets. One thing's for sure, biochemistry and physiology don't lie. This new (to me) body of evidence started making a lot of sense, it all seemed so logical, far more logical than the mainstream nutrition story. I wondered why I had never come across this work before now. Next up, I came across the brilliant work of Gary Taubes[2] and Nina Teicholz[3], who both eloquently exposed the politics of the nutrition story, and in particular the influence of the food and pharmaceutical industries. And finally, I got wind of the noise being made by Professor Tim Noakes (my Cape Town exercise physiology lecturer who passionately stressed the importance of carbs and high carb diets for athletes way back when). When I heard his story and consequent nutrition change of heart, I knew there had to be something to it. You see, he is not new to controversy. He was instrumental in changing the face of fluid guidelines for ultra-endurance athletes several years back from a precise mls of fluid per hour instruction to a "drink to thirst" guideline. This was largely due to the increasing incidence of hyponatraemia in these athletes who followed the mainstream fluid guidelines. Hyponatremia is a potentially fatal condition of low blood sodium levels; it occurs when athletes drink too much fluid during their ultra-endurance events and essentially "dissolve" the sodium in their bloodstream. The "drink to thirst" guideline flew in the face of mainstream fluid and hydration guidelines, but despite being contentious at the time, he was spot-on with moving the science forward. Eventually the guidelines changed at the level of the ACSM (American College of Sports Medicine), and hyponatremia in these

147

athletes virtually disappeared. So when Prof Noakes started making noise about carbs and fat, and health and disease, no matter how controversial it was, I knew there was bound to be more to the story.

Enter... Hyperinsulinemia

The term hyperinsulinemia is no longer just a great hangman word to me, it now sits at the core of my understanding, and dietary management of Type 2 diabetes. For the last several years, I have had the privilege of working with ex-Ph.D student and pharmacist (now *Dr)* Catherine Crofts and the legendary, late Dr Joseph Kraft (US pathologist). I was introduced to Dr Kraft's life's work of insulin curves, Kraft patterns and hyperinsulinemia, a condition that is now being considered an independent risk factor for metabolic disease rather than just a symptom of insulin resistance.[4, 5] During this time, my understanding of the extent to which chronically raised levels of insulin damages the body, along with the discovery that glucose curves can be totally normal despite insulin levels being screamingly high, has revolutionised my dietetic practice[6]. My new focus for diabetes management is not just about managing blood sugar any which way necessary and "patching" food around medications, it is now about tending to the underlying problem. Blood sugar alone has stepped aside in many cases and made way for the real villain, insulin.

The cornerstone of mainstream dietetic guidance for diabetes, as you would typically find in the hospital system in New Zealand (and I assume across the globe), is to consume a diet of at least 250 g of carbs each day (or 45-65% of total energy) with very little fat[7]. It usually includes advice to eat five to six times a day, with carbs as the dominant nutrient at each meal. This is a system that has clearly not yet acknowledged the science (or developed the appropriate diagnostics) around insulin resistance or hyperinsulinemia. It's a system that expects the overweight diabetic to rid themselves of excess body fat while their high levels of insulin (a storage hormone) prevents exactly that from occurring. Instead, any effort to lose excess fat is attempted in a low fat, calorie-scrimping, over-exercising, hunger-managing manner. It's a non-sustainable damage control system with a modus operandi of medications-first, food-second that just does not address the real problem. It's no wonder the pharmaceutical industry is booming.

Tiptoeing into clinical practice...

When you come to the realisation that what you have believed and practised for your entire career might be wrong, and then do a 180 degree flip and go against all your dietetic peers, it doesn't make for an easy transition. In fact, for the first couple of months, when confusion preceded my awakening, I seriously contemplated changing my profession. The problem was that with my new body of knowledge, I simply couldn't let it go and return to business as usual, or abandon the nutrition ship completely. So, after reforming my own diet, and feeling satisfied that I had read enough to be convinced, I started to implement this in clinical practice. It wasn't so much the reduction in carbs that I had a problem with, but more so the addition of fat. The first consultation with my new "hat" felt wrong, in fact I can still feel the cold shivers work their way down my spine when I recall telling a client to stock full fat milk, yoghurt and cheese, and replace their industrial seed oil-based margarine with butter. But as the continuous stream of success stories rolled in, I became even more convinced that this is how it should have been all along, and is for certain, the way forward in nutrition. This list shows many of the benefits that my clients have reported after incorporating the LCHF philosophy into their lives:

Weight loss (if needed)	Clearer skin
Reduced joint pain	Improved moods
Less bloated / wind	Reduced brain fog
Reduced PMS symptoms	Clearer mind
Reduced gut issues	Improved lipid profile
Reduced muscle soreness	Improved concentration
Stable blood sugar	Increased satiety
Reduced medications	Increased energy
Reduced heart palpitations	Improved psoriasis condition
Improved sleep	Improved eyesight

In my 20 years of private practice, it is only during the last 5 years of practising as an LCHF dietitian that I have heard clients report such an extensive range of positive outcomes, just from altering their diet. As an academic, I firmly believe that evidence from trials is important to inform practice, but so often you see practice leading the way and research catching up. As a practitioner, I think that these outcomes speak for themselves.

Spreading the "whole" LCHF message ...

When LCHF eating comes under attack – which is more often than not, it appears that our critics constantly seem to get it wrong. It's often described as 'high protein', 'severely restricted', 'a fad diet' and 'no-carb' – none of which is correct. Our critics also say that we are going to confuse the public as they might only hear half the message.

So, to get the right messages and the whole story out there at a level beyond the one-to-one nutrition consulting clinic, three of us got together and wrote a book: Myself, AUT Professor Grant Schofield and UK-born chef, Craig Rodger, founder of the first official LCHF restaurant in Auckland, NZ. We called the book "What The Fat?" Abbreviated to WTF?[8] – for obvious reasons! Covering the science and the practice around what we called low carb, *healthy* fat (LCHF), consumers can now read the full story, and hopefully avoid any confusion with mixed, or half messages. Our mission in writing the book was to get the right messages out there and of course to help people make changes in their nutrition behaviours and lifestyle, for good! The content of the book is centred around 10 rules, which I've summarised for you here:

Rule number 1: *Go low "HI"*	Replace processed foods with stuff that was recently alive – foods low in the human interference (HI) factor. Real, whole, actual food is the foundation of the LCHF lifestyle.
Rule number 2: *Cut the carbs down, not out.*	There is a spectrum of "low carb" and just how low you go depends on your personal tolerance to carbs, or degree of insulin resistance. A perfect place to start is to cut down on the processed carbs.

Rule number 3: *Virtuous vegetables*	Vegetables are good for you. Eat lots of them, at each meal if possible. The good news is you can add fats such as olive oil or butter to make them taste even better.
Rule number 4: *Make fat your friend*	For us, it's 'low carb, *healthy* fat'. This doesn't mean drowning every meal in cream and eating blocks of butter just because you now know eating saturated fat *in the context of whole food* is ok. We know that monounsaturated fats and polyunsaturated fats (omega 3, that is) are beneficial so mix it up and get over your fat phobia.
Rule number 5: *Put protein in its place*	You need protein for life, but once you have more than your body needs, it gets converted into sugars by the liver. LCHF is not a high-protein diet. Many people stall in their progress because they are overdoing the protein.
Rule number 6: *Eat on cue*	The whole point of LCHF is that your body will now be able to send and receive the messages it needs to stay in shape, to tell you when you are full, and to energise you.
Rule number 7: *Sort your support*	Other people matter. Surround yourself with helpers, ask for support, and don't be afraid to request exactly what you want when you are out and about. Yes, it feels odd to order a burger without the bun the first time, but you will be amazed at how much people will help someone on a life mission.
Rule number 8: *Diligence, not effort*	Relying on your "won't power" (effort) – like avoiding the chocolate cookies in your pantry – is futile. Instead, rely on being organised and having a ready supply of the right foods around you (diligence) in the first place.

Rule number 9: *Adopt the "3-meal" rule*	You, like us, are human. Humans make mistakes. We do, and we expect you will fall off the wagon. That's okay as long as we can help you jump back on again. We run the 3-meal rule: there are 3 meals a day, 21 meals in a week. Let's get most of them right, knowing that three meals off the wagon a week is okay.
Rule number 10: *It's not just about the food*	News flash from the prof and Dr Obvious: other things also affect your health – exercise, booze and cigarettes, drugs, stress, sleep, and much more. You need to figure out how these fit (or don't fit) into the LCHF lifestyle.

In this undefined space of LCHF eating, the devil is certainly in the detail when it comes to exactly how many grams of carbs, protein and fat you should eat. LCHF has a wide spectrum, and your specifics will depend on your own unique set of circumstances and goals. The bottom line is that it's all about altering the current highly processed, packaged way of eating to one which is whole-food based, and constantly chipping away at changing behaviours so that it becomes a life-long journey. My philosophy is that if you truly eat whole food it will work out to be LCHF.

Celebrating successes

While I have hundreds of success stories, here are two of our precious diabetes case studies that appear in our WTF? book[8].

First up is pilot, Gary Bridger. Gary came to see me in my consulting clinic, panicked by a recent diagnosis of prediabetes. Several weeks later, after following my advice and converting his family and many friends to LCHF along the way, he successfully reversed his diagnosis. That was 3 years ago, and he has still managed to keep it at bay. Gary is a total champion, and I still have contact with him today. He is still enjoying the LCHF lifestyle and it is clear that he has changed his eating habits, for life. He still sends me text messages with pictures of his LCHF meals, and forwards on emails from people that he has converted along with their success stories. Gary's story is one of many that makes my work as an LCHF dietitian totally rewarding.

Here's Gary's story:

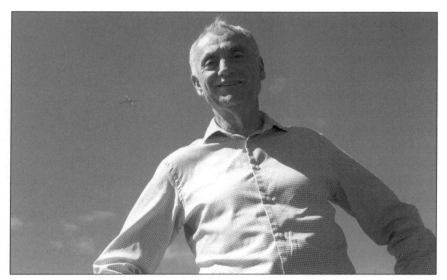

Diabetes averted: 17 kg weight loss without effort. Gary Bridger, 55, Air New Zealand A320 captain

The triggers that led me to LCHF were a steady increase in weight and a rising blood sugar count whenever I did my commercial pilot licence medical. Pilots are generally very health conscious. Our continued employment depends on it. If you end up with diabetes, that's the end of being a pilot.

A fellow pilot and long-term friend convinced me of the perils of excessive sugar in our diet, so I started off by drastically cutting down on sugar. The results were a 6 kg drop in weight, but little change to the rising blood sugar levels. I was perilously close to Type 2 diabetes, and to being unemployed.

It was only then that I visited Dr Caryn Zinn, who put me on a carb-restricted, healthy-fat diet to lower my blood sugar levels and further reduce my weight. She also got me to download an app for my iPhone for tracking my carb and protein intake. Following Caryn's eating plan, the results were immediate and dramatic. After three months eating the low-carb way, I had lost another 11 kg (17 kg total) and my HbA1c blood sugar control reading had gone from "pre-diabetic" to "normal".

I have been absolutely delighted with the results and am committed to LCHF eating long term. Fortunately, I have had excellent support from my wife and family, who have also embraced the new way of eating. This whole experience has been a huge benefit to me. Just to have my weight and blood sugar levels under control gives me not only the security of employment, but I also feel much more energetic than before. Because I have benefited so much, I have continued to spread the word amongst fellow pilots, family and friends. Many have taken up the challenge and all have had similar results.

The hardest part of LCHF eating for me was finding suitable meals at work and away from home. Many cafés simply don't offer LCHF options, but with a little imagination you can adapt. For example, a Caesar salad without the croutons is a good solution, or a burger and salad and just leave the bun and fries. I also take small packets of nuts with me for snacks to tide me over until I can find suitable meal options.

For favourite foods, I do enjoy breakfast with eggs, bacon or sausage, mushrooms and green vegetables for a good start to the day. That breakfast for me is the key and keeps me going nicely until lunchtime. For lunch, always a salad at home, and the salad bar at the Auckland airport is an oasis for LCHF eating! Family evening meal favourites include roast lamb and ratatouille with cauliflower mashed with butter, and parmesan cheese. Other favourites are lasagne with sliced courgettes instead of pasta and "potato top" pie with mashed cauliflower instead of potato. We have been eating more fish than before and, of course, more "above ground" vegetables. I have also been cooking Malaysian (our favourite ethnic food) chicken or fish curries with plenty of added vegetables and cauliflower rice instead of conventional rice – divine!

Next I want to introduce you to my longtime friend, Trish. Trish has been a Type 1 diabetic for as long as I've known her, and despite my "best practice" advice to her over the years, she has just never been able to keep both her weight and her blood sugars totally under control. Here's Trish's story:

When I was diagnosed with diabetes 25 years ago, it was a bit of a shock as I ate well and was pretty fit. I didn't know much about diabetes, but my attitude was to just get on with things and lead a normal life. I thought, "Well, I just have to keep eating healthily and stay fit for the rest of my life."

In recent years, I have moved along with technology and switched to an insulin pump. I track my blood sugar and program the pump to deliver the required insulin (which I can't produce myself – that's what a Type 1 diabetic is) to maintain my blood sugar at between 6 and 6.4 mmol/l.

Part of the problem with being a Type 1 diabetic is you get "hypos", which happen when you fail to match your carb intake and insulin properly; that is, you eat too few carbs and have more insulin in your body than you need. This results in low blood sugar, which can have severe consequences if you're not careful, as hypos can lead to blacking out. One time, I was out swimming by myself in the ocean, training for a half ironman, when I had a hypo. Luckily, I was close to shore and was rescued by someone walking on the beach. I tried to get back in the water, but he pulled me out again and called the paramedics. I don't want to think about what could have happened if he had not been there.

The big advantage I have noticed from LCHF is that even if my blood sugar goes low, the effect isn't too severe. I am much more "hypo-proof" on LCHF. Other advantages include:

- I have effortlessly dropped several kilos

- My HbA1c has dropped from 8.8% to 6.2%

- My insulin use is down by 30% (from 30 units per day to 21)

- My blood cholesterol results are awesome – they were awesome before, but importantly they are still awesome, even though I eat loads of fat

- I have heaps of energy and feel great

One thing which helped along the way is that this became a social thing with my friends. We were all giving it a go. So going LCHF was pretty cool and we were (are) all into working out how many carbs were in different foods and what some yummy foods to eat were. It's been fun and it's really cool that LCHF suits my style of eating, my health and my diabetes.

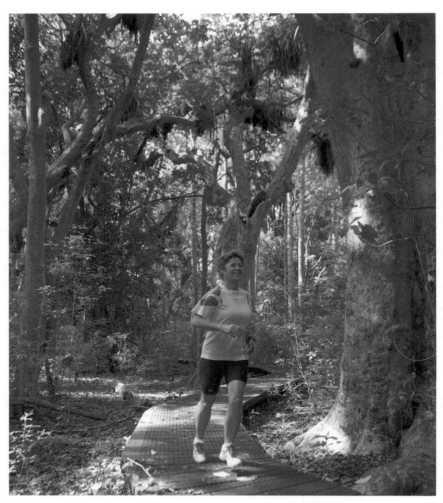

Proof LCHF helps Type 1 Diabetes. Trish Bradbury, 55, University Lecturer

Stifling the LCHF message... "Down Under"

"Going against the grain" (so-to-speak) of mainstream nutrition for many health professionals has certainly not been smooth sailing, particularly Down Under – Australia and New Zealand. In Australia, two dieticians have been deregistered, undoubtedly due to their work relating to LCHF eating, and a prominent orthopedic surgeon "silenced" as a result of his advocacy work in the whole food, LCHF domain. Perhaps it's a Southern Hemisphere issue as we all know about the longstanding three year "Nutrition trial of the century" that Prof Tim Noakes has faced.

On a personal front, I have been spending a fair bit of time over the last few years providing response after response to the New Zealand Dietitians Board for formal complaints about my work related to LCHF, including my social media presence in this space. Several complaints came from more "established" dieticians, others from colleagues with which I have always had respectful and positive working relationships, which is a little disappointing. My last complaint was on behalf of the DAA, the Dietetics Association of Australia. It was a three-pager and listed a collection of my supposed wrongdoings – many of which contained factual errors.

On a positive note, the New Zealand Dietitians Board has followed process well and has indicated that it is satisfied with the safety of my practice and finds no reason to progress any of the complaints to de-registration. Without knowing what tomorrow will bring, I have been free of formal complaints now for almost 2 years and am starting to feel like the true message is getting out there in a safe way, both to my dietetic peers as well as to the community. I have also become a mentor to many dieticians around the globe who wish to learn more about the ins and outs of LCHF nutrition. All in all, it's been a challenging, yet rewarding few years which I would never change if I could have it repeated. I'm confident that the whole food, LCHF lifestyle will be the way of the future, and I'm privileged to be a part of leading the way towards it.

Dr Caryn Zinn, Ph.D

@carynzinn
carynzinn.co.nz
What The Fat?: Fat's IN: Sugar's OUT Practical guide and recipes, The Real Food Publishing Company 2015
What The Fat?: Sport Performance Leaner, Fitter, Faster on Low Carb, Healthy Fat. The Real Food Publishing Company 2016. (For more information, check out the details here: https://whatthefatbook.com/)

Chapter Nine

Why and how should we monitor glucose levels?

By Dr Neville Wellington

In 2011 and 2012 I was fortunate enough to do a postgraduate diploma in diabetes through the University of Cardiff, which, quite frankly, changed my professional life. I did it because I realised that I knew so little about diabetes, even though I had been treating patients for the past 15 years, and was frustrated that I did not seem to be making much progress. I was certain that the knowledge to free patients from this scourge existed and I just needed to tap into that knowledge and learn the tricks of the trade, so to speak. During the 2 years, I was exposed to about 600 journal articles per module, a number of textbooks, and many discussions with fellow students. It was thoroughly enlightening, but at no point did I discover the secrets to 'cure' or reverse diabetes. In retrospect, the most significant aspects I learnt were around the dietary recommendations, and more particularly, how carbohydrates increase a patient's glucose levels, and how glucose causes inflammatory changes in cells. By the end of the course I was strongly under the impression that diabetes is a progressive, relentless disease and all we had were fairly inadequate medications to try and control it. Eventually all patients with Type 2 diabetes would need insulin and this was just a matter of time. Glucose is essential for life and there was no talk of reducing carbohydrate intakes, only really of insulin to carbohydrate ratios. You just have to match your carbohydrates to your medication and all would be fine, or so I read.

In 2012, I received a letter from Professor Tim Noakes, which detailed the recent journey he had been on into the low carbohydrate world. At the time I was so involved in my studies that I paid little attention to it, but did wonder why he, who was someone I had always respected, would be going against, not only his own wisdom, but the prevailing conventional wisdom. However, as I continued my studies, I began to see that what he was advocating actually made sense from a physiological

159

point of view. Added to this, I began to see patients who had started to adopt a low carbohydrate lifestyle and who were achieving greater success with their diabetes, and who really inspired me to learn more about low carbohydrate lifestyles. Professor Noakes had sent us a list of books and articles he had read and I read through those, once I had completed my studies. I have since then continued to research this more deeply and encouraged my patients to apply this lifestyle to their diabetes. Many have achieved excellent improvements in their diabetes control and been able to maintain this for a number of years now.

So, as I have been treating patients this way for the past four years I have been refining and developing my approach and have found that there are a number of factors that help patients be successful in controlling their disease. These are:

- Following a low carbohydrate lifestyle and increasing their own knowledge of what this entails;

- Being guided by a doctor who is prepared to be open to this lifestyle;

- Monitoring their glucose levels in a structured manner;

- Having a team who can support them, such as a diabetes educator, a diabetes nurse, an informed dietician, and specialists who will care for complications;

- Having excellent and positive family support.

While all of these are important, I would like in this chapter to concentrate on glucose monitoring, as that gives us the hard data as to whether patients are achieving success in their disease. I'll look at this under two headings: 'Why should we monitor glucose levels' and 'How should we monitor glucose levels'.

Why should we monitor glucose levels?

At the outset I would like to explain what is normal for non-diabetic patients. While I understand that there is controversy about what is 'normal', and there is no doubt that the cardiovascular damage caused by high glucose levels is on a continuum, we do need some reference points. Most guidelines around the world define glucose levels as follows[1]:

Normal fasting levels <5.6 mmol/l*

After meal readings (90-120 mins after the start of the meal) <7.8 mmol/l

Normal HbA1c levels <5.7% or 37.7 mmol/mol.

Over the years I have tested hundreds of non-diabetic patients' glucose levels, and they usually fall in this range. From this I have also seen that a normal pre-meal level is between 4-5.6 mmol/l. Studies on cardiovascular disease and corresponding HbA1c levels have also shown a linear increase in cardiovascular disease as HbA1c levels increase.[2-6] One study has even shown that cardiovascular disease rates are at their lowest below an HbA1c level of 4.6%.[4] We should, therefore, as far as is safely possible, aim towards normal glucose levels in all patients and not accept the higher levels that guidelines give us, as we try to reduce the risks of diabetes to as low as possible. This can only be achieved by following careful low carbohydrate lifestyles and with careful monitoring.

As I noted earlier, glucose monitoring helps to confirm if we are being successful in treating our diabetes, but there are other reasons to monitor glucose levels regularly. **First**, we need to ensure that patients are safe, especially in terms of hypoglycemic spells. Any change in diet or medication necessitates more regular testing to ensure that glucose levels do not fall too low. In most cases patients should reduce or even stop hypoglycemic medications when they change to low carbohydrate lifestyles. This is often one of the biggest reasons why patients will lose confidence in low carbohydrate lifestyles, and give up. **Secondly**, for those taking insulin, or any medication that stimulates insulin release from the pancreas, monitoring glucose levels will help to ensure that the doses they are taking are correct. **Thirdly**, (and I believe the most important reason) is to monitor

---

* To convert mmol/l to mg/dL multiply by 18.

161

the glucose response to meals. I have seen that those who eat low carbohydrate meals are able to control the change in their glucose levels far easier; that is the rise from the pre-meal reading to the post-meal reading. The lower the rise the better the control and this leads to better long term results. I aim for a rise of not more than about 1.7 mmol/l, although if a patient eats less than 10 g of carbohydrates in a meal, the rise may be negligible. Ultimately, it becomes obvious that diabetes is controlled (or even reversed) one meal at a time.

By monitoring carefully, patients are able to assess their progress and determine for themselves what they can and cannot eat. I often tell patients that they don't need to believe what I tell them, but rather see the evidence for themselves by monitoring their glucose levels. Usually this confirms what I have explained to them. Many times I have seen new patients who have done this very well, and have proven for themselves, through glucose monitoring, that low carbohydrate lifestyles are a realistic and safe option. They just come to me to help support and monitor their progress. Richard Bernstein discovered this when he started monitoring his glucose levels many years ago and was able to control his diabetes and prevent further complications.[7]

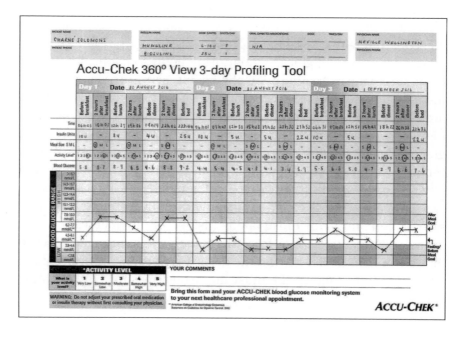

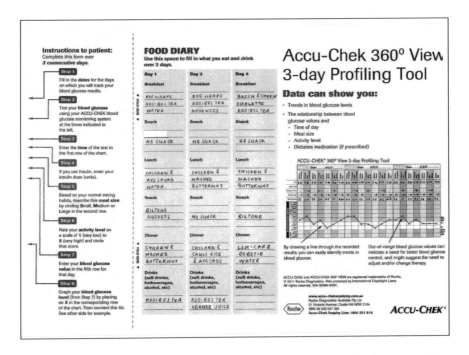

To help one understand why some readings may be high, it is really important to understand how many carbohydrates (measured in grams) are in certain foods. I train all my patients in carbohydrate counting and teach them to read labels. To be successful at achieving good glucose levels patients do need to be able to calculate how many grams of carbohydrates they are eating per meal.

How should we monitor glucose levels?

Glucose levels are monitored most commonly by using handheld glucose meters (or glucometers). There are many on the market and all patients with diabetes should have a working meter. They are readily available, although the cost of strips can vary quite considerably. Continuous glucose monitors (CGM) are fast becoming available, and have the advantage of less finger pricking, but are very expensive at this stage. My hope is that all patients will have easier access to CGM, even if only for a few months to help them to establish a new lifestyle.

I see patients at all stages of their diabetes journey. Often I see patients who have had diabetes for many years and when I ask them about their monitoring, invariably it is very haphazard. Many patients with Type 2 diabetes only monitor their early morning readings, and occasionally at other times when they are not feeling so well. Unfortunately, all this tells them is that they are diabetic (glucose levels above 7 mmol/l are diagnostic of diabetes), but it doesn't help in changing their lifestyles or their medication. Quite frankly, haphazard testing in this way is 'pain with very little gain'!

Glucose monitoring must be structured if it is going to help improve control. This means that, ideally all meals should be monitored before and after eating. Studies show that meal time glucose levels spike at about 60 to 90 minutes after the start of the meal, so the glucose levels should be checked at this stage[8]. Sometimes it may be necessary to check a few times after the meal to confirm when the spike occurs. In general, fluid meals (like shakes) will spike quicker (around 30 minutes), whereas fat containing meals may take longer to spike (around 120 to 150 minutes). The aim, as mentioned earlier, is to have readings before meals of 4-6 mmol/l and post meals of less than 7.7 mmol/l.

Almost all glucometers can be downloaded onto computers and it is useful to download the software. I have almost all the software of the various meters, so I do ask all patients to bring in their meters to each consultation. This is particularly helpful to see regular patterns (e.g. low readings in the mornings may indicate an overuse of insulin) and also to see if patients are testing correctly. However, it is even more helpful if patients record these readings in a diary along with the meals eaten and medication or insulin taken. There are many glucose diaries available and I do give out those that the glucometer companies produce. Many patients make up their own spreadsheets and I find these very helpful, as they contain the most information. This should then be reviewed by their doctor. With this data I can quickly see where patients are struggling with meals, or need to reduce (usually) or increase (seldom) their medication. In general, it becomes very obvious that 'lows' (hypoglycemia) are caused by too much medication, and 'highs' (hyperglycemia) are caused by too much carbohydrate. When readings are very variable (i.e. big swings from 'lows' to 'highs' or vice versa), then both medications and carbohydrates need to be lowered proportionally. Each meal becomes a research project; if post meal levels are high, it's important to analyse the reasons for this. Sometimes, it's something new you are eating, other times you just did not realise how many carbohydrates are in foods that you regularly eat (e.g. tomatoes).

Once patients, especially those with Type 2 diabetes, have stabilised their readings as close to normal as possible, then testing can be reduced to one or two meals only per day. This could take one to two months if patients are very committed. Ideally I hope to see patients change their lifestyles to such an extent that they are able to be on minimum or no medication and have normalised their HbA1c levels. Then they will be able to live 'normal' lives, although always following a low carbohydrate lifestyle.

Conclusions

What I have written about is the ideal. Some patients are able to incorporate this into their lives quite quickly, and improve their diabetes control in a few months. Others find it more difficult, due to family, work and social constraints, or even just embarrassment around their disease. Many, who have been diabetic for years, have to unlearn their old habits, which can seem overwhelming at times. My advice is to get started with even one meal a day. Every bit of information is useful. As success increases so it becomes easier to test more and inspire yourself to improving your health. No matter how far you have gone down the wrong road, you can always turn around. I have been blessed to see many patients achieve great success in this and they have inspired me to keep helping others. While lifestyle changes are the cornerstone to controlling diabetes, glucose monitoring is the tool that will confirm that the changes are working.

Dr Neville Wellington

@nevillewellingt

Chapter Ten

Is Type 2 diabetes just too much sugar?
What happens when it's cut?

by Dr David Unwin

Imagine that you are a family doctor, caring for a close knit community of about 9,000 people for 30 years. During that time, despite many and varied efforts, you watch the two epidemics of obesity and Type 2 diabetes take a terrible grip on your patients. Nothing you do seems to help – despite the fact that you are prescribing ever more medication, doing more blood tests and every day warning your patients about the urgent need to lose weight. It feels hopeless, despairing, but then two patients, one book and a single fact change everything. A eureka moment occurs, which enables you at last to help many patients with the two epidemics of modern life: diabetes and obesity. And without using lifelong medication.

That doctor was me! And now I can't let it go. A sensible voice says I could be biased, or possibly just showing off, that this is all part of my desperation to make a difference at the end of my career. After weighing these possibilities in mind I still conclude that so much disease, disability and unhappiness is possibly all a result of just too much sugar.

After I joined my practice in 1986, we did a survey of our patients with Type 2 diabetes (T2DM); there were just 57 cases. In 'the olden days' we called this either 'sugar diabetes' or 'maturity onset diabetes' to reflect the fact that T2DM usually developed in patients in their mid-sixties or older, and that sugar was understood to be part of its causation. At that time, there were no patients with T2DM under the age of 50. Now, 30 years on, we have 21 patients (with an average body weight of 111.5 kg or 246 pounds) under 50. The youngest is 34. I have also seen a more than six fold increase in the prevalence of diagnosed diabetes with well over 400 patients now having T2DM. Something has changed. It cannot be my patients' genes – not in one generation – but rather a changed environment acting upon a genetic predisposition. Four years ago, I had no idea why this was, or that anything could be done to halt the tide of this disabling condition and the associated epidemic of obesity. Yet there just had to be a cause for all of this.

Two patients, one book and a single fact change everything.

Patient 1: Reversal/remission of T2DM following weight loss.

For many years, I had looked after a very overweight patient (115 kg BMI 40), with moderate diabetes, needing a high dose of the drug metformin to maintain even poor diabetes control (HbA1c 65 mmol/mol). The patient started experiencing vomiting and abdominal pains, which, despite specialist opinions and scans, went on for nine months causing a 50 kg weight loss. I wondered if the vomiting could be a side effect of treatment, and within two weeks of stopping her metformin, the patient felt miraculously better. A few months later, it transpired that the diabetes had been reversed; the HbA1c was quite normal at 35 mmol/mol. The patient felt so much better off the metformin, but over the next two years she was back up to 115 kg and once again had a HbA1c of 65 mmol/mol.

This case taught me that diabetes was potentially reversible with weight loss and that the diabetes drug, metformin, was not always the best treatment.

Patient 2: First low-carb patient to come off medication.

I was worried because one of my patients with diabetes was not ordering her diabetes medications as usual or coming to clinic. Concerned, I rang her personally and invited her in – only to discover that, following a three stone weight loss, she was unrecognisable! Full of apologies she explained "I daren't tell you what I've done as I know you will be so annoyed." It turned out that she had joined the low carbohydrate forum of Diabetes.co.uk and given up bread, rice and potatoes. When her blood test results came back, despite no medication, her diabetes was in remission. Her blood pressure was also so much better.

This taught me that a low carbohydrate diet was an option for people with T2DM. I was so humbled by the fact that she was scared of telling me about this, I was determined to find out more and so joined the forum myself. At the time, the low carbohydrate community had been ridiculed so often by health care professionals that the forum members struggled to believe that I could be trusted. As a result, within days I was removed from the forum as a likely 'troll.' This had a profound effect on me, as a health professional who had devoted his life to trying to help others. There were so many individuals doing incredibly well and yet they did not feel able to trust a doctor to work with them. I became determined to find out more about the basis of this approach.

One book: Escape The Diet Trap by Dr John Briffa

Dr John Briffa, in his excellent book, introduced me to some nutritional principles. Briffa made the point that, while fats contain the essential vitamins A, D, E & K, sugar represents 'empty calories'. If T2DM is largely about sugar, why should people with diabetes take in the 'concentrated sugar' that is in starchy foods such as bread, pasta or rice?

This book explained matters so well that, in January 2013, I bought 20 copies to give to interested patients with diabetes. I asked them to give me feedback. Within weeks I got my feedback: stories of 'feeling more alive'; not being hungry; the experience of painless weight loss. By this time the practice nurse, Heather, my wife Jen and I had joined them on a low carbohydrate diet and we knew just what they meant.

And the Fact: The glycaemic index of table sugar is 65 and brown bread is 74.[1]

I read this in the British Medical Journal. I was so incredulous and thought that there must be some mistake. Surely bread could *not* have a worse effect on blood glucose than table sugar, and 'healthy' brown bread at that? I usually told people with diabetes to avoid sugar, but that bread was OK. I checked the International tables for the glycaemic index and found, to my amazement, that the figures were correct.

The glycaemic index of a food is defined as the area under the blood glucose response curve, measured in the two hours following consumption of that food. The blood glucose response curve captures the peak in blood glucose and the time period over which the blood glucose was raised. Glucose (being pure glucose) itself is assigned a glycaemic index (GI) of 100 and then all foods are measured relative to this score of 100.

The GI score of a particular food tells us, in effect, how much glucose gets into the blood stream, in the two hour period after consuming that particular food, relative to consuming pure glucose itself. The GI number for different foods is annoyingly rarely the same from two different sources, but the numbers are generally close enough.

The GI throws up some surprises. Table sugar, for example, has a GI of 65. That gives table sugar a lower GI than brown bread (74) and baked potato (85).

The discovery and understanding of the glycaemic index made me consider: So perhaps starchy foods are a concentrated source of glucose?

Putting the pieces together

So now the pieces were in place.

- Diabetes was potentially reversible with weight loss.

- The diabetes drug metformin was not always the best treatment.

- The glycaemic index of table sugar is 65, and brown bread is 74 (worse).

- The low carbohydrate diet was an option for people with T2DM.

- If T2DM is largely about sugar, why should people with diabetes take in the 'concentrated sugar' that is in starchy foods such as bread, pasta or rice?

Our general medical practice used the advice in Dr John Briffa's book as a basis. To this we added i) information about the predicted effect on post-prandial (after eating) blood glucose from the glycaemic index and ii) feedback from the first 20 patients interested in trying a lower carbohydrate diet. Our basic diet and information sheet was thus developed – this is shared in full below.

T2DM Advice sheet for patients[2]

So what should I eat to control Diabetes or Pre-diabetes?

Reduce starchy carbs a lot (remember they are just concentrated sugar). If possible cut out the 'White Stuff' like bread, pasta, rice – though porridge, new potatoes and oat cakes in moderation may be fine. Sugar – cut it out altogether, although it will be in the blueberries, strawberries and raspberries you are allowed to eat freely. Cakes and biscuits are a mixture of sugar and starch that make it almost impossible to avoid food cravings; they just make you hungrier!!

All green veg/salads are fine – eat as much as you can. So that you still eat a good big dinner try substituting veg such as broccoli, courgettes or green beans for your mash, pasta or rice – still covering them with your gravy, bolognese or curry! Tip: try home-made soup – it can be taken to work for lunch and microwaved. Mushrooms, tomatoes, and onions can be included in this.

Fruit is trickier; some have too much sugar in and can set those carb cravings off. All berries are great and can be eaten freely; blueberries, raspberries, strawberries, apples and pears too, but not tropical fruits like bananas, oranges, grapes, mangoes or pineapples.

Proteins such as in meat, eggs, fish – particularly oily fish such as salmon, mackerel or tuna – are fine and can be eaten freely. Plain full fat yoghurt makes a good breakfast with the berries.

Processed meats such as bacon, ham, sausages or salami are not as healthy and should only be eaten in moderation.

Fats (yes, fats can be fine in moderation): olive oil is very useful, butter may be tastier than margarine and could be better for you! Coconut oil is great for stir fries. Four essential vitamins A, D, E and K are only found in some fats or oils. Please avoid margarine, corn oil and vegetable oil. Beware 'low fat' foods. They often have sugar or sweeteners added to make them palatable.

Full fat mayonnaise and pesto are definitely on!!

Cheese: only in moderation – it's a very calorific mixture of fat and protein.

Snacks: avoid. But un-salted nuts such as almonds or walnuts are great to stave off hunger. The occasional treat of strong dark chocolate 70% or more in small quantity is allowed.

EATING LOTS OF VEG WITH PROTEIN AND FATS LEAVES YOU PROPERLY FULL in a way that lasts.

Finally, about sweeteners and what to drink – sweeteners have been proven to tease your brain into being even more hungry making weight loss almost impossible – drink tea, coffee, and water or herb teas. I'm afraid alcoholic drinks are full of carbohydrate – for example, beer is almost 'liquid toast' hence the beer belly!! Perhaps the odd glass of red wine wouldn't be too bad if it doesn't make you get hungry afterwards – or just plain water with a slice of lemon.

Where to get more info?

A book – 'Escape the diet trap' by Dr John Briffa (2013). Well researched and easy to read.

Internet – Google 'about.com low carb diet' for loads more info and recipes, or look into the closely related PALEO DIET; also Google 'diabetes.co.uk forum low carb' for contact, recipes and hints.

BEFORE YOU START get an accurate weight and measure your waist, re-weigh and measure once a week to see how you are doing and ask for help if problems or little progress is being made – GO ON DO IT!!!

No need to weigh food or calorie count.

Quite unlike all the diets I had advised in the 25 years before this, we found that if patients understood the principles of the lower carbohydrate diet, and, importantly were committed to change, there was really no need to weigh portions or calorie count. One patient, Elizabeth (weight loss of over 20 kg sustained for three years and ongoing) put it rather well, *'previously with diets all the weighing and measuring is a constant reminder of the fact you are on a diet. Diets are things you are on, and then come off, this is more of a new and permanent lifestyle'.*

A third epidemic: non-alcoholic fatty liver disease (NAFLD): Is sugar implicated here too?

While working with the first twenty patients, who were having regular blood tests, I noticed very surprising and rapid improvements in liver function, particularly in the levels of a liver enzyme, gamma-glutamyl transferase (GGT). I had previously been worried by how many of my patients had abnormal liver function. Out of 4,753 practice patients, having liver function blood tests done over three years, a shocking 1,153 (24%) had an abnormal GGT result. I have already mentioned two epidemics – diabetes and obesity – well there is a third epidemic just as large, but rarely mentioned, and that is non-alcoholic fatty liver disease (NAFLD).

Many of you may have heard of "fatty liver". This non-alcoholic form now affects 20% of the developed world and is a very common cause of a raised GGT result.[3] NAFLD seems to be linked with diabetes and heart disease. The famous Framingham Heart Study, for example, provided evidence that individuals in the highest GGT quartile experienced a 67% increase in cardiovascular disease incidence. This result was informed by 19 years of follow up in 3,451 individuals.[4]

There are two forms of fatty liver: Alcoholic and Non-alcoholic fatty liver disease (NAFLD). Even with a microscope a doctor cannot tell the difference, which is interesting. Often when presented with abnormal liver function blood-tests doctors may assume (often wrongly) that the patient drinks too much alcohol:

172

"Mrs Jones when you say it's a 'small sherry once a month' – I wonder if you are sure it's not just a bit more?"

It is interesting that excess alcohol and dietary sugar seem to affect the liver in such similar ways. This has resulted in some of my patients with abnormal liver function suffering from the prejudice that their abnormal liver function was a result of alcohol abuse and yet, as we demonstrated, often this was not the case.

Our published study, "Raised GGT levels, Diabetes and NAFLD: Is dietary carbohydrate a link?"[5] suggested that reducing sugar and carbs in the diet could have a dramatic effect in improving liver function, for people who report low alcohol consumption; a hitherto little reported benefit of the low-carb diet on top of the effects for obesity and diabetes.

In his 2012 Banting lecture, Professor Roy Taylor of Newcastle University UK[6] reported that abnormal liver function tests and NAFLD often predate the onset of diabetes by many years; *"Before diagnosis of Type 2 diabetes, there is a long silent scream from the liver".*

In 2009, a systematic review and meta-analysis of 18 prospective, population-based studies, including more than 280,000 patient years of follow up, showed that mildly raised serum liver enzyme results were independent, long-term predictors of incident T2DM.[7]

There is also evidence linking abnormal liver function with central obesity, as well as T2DM.[8] This adds to my suspicion stated earlier that these three modern epidemics – obesity, T2DM and Non-alcoholic fatty liver disease – share a common cause. This suggests that they may also have a shared remedy – the radical reduction of dietary refined carbs and sugar.

Our own study results on liver function have been impressive.[9] We looked at a case series of 69 patients on a low sugar, low carbohydrate diet with abnormal liver function. After an average of 13 months on the diet (as shown on the "Advice sheet"), the following results were achieved:

- There was an average 46% improvement in liver blood tests (GGT);

- There was an average 8.8 kg weight loss (from an average 98 kg to 89 kg);

- Diabetes control improved with HbA1c down from 52.4 mmol/mol to 42.4 mmol/mol. This moved the average person from the description "diabetic" to very nearly "normal/ nondiabetic";

- Average total cholesterol levels fell from 5.7 mmol/L to 5.3 mmol/L. This was despite a diet higher in butter, eggs, olive oil and other healthy fats;

- Blood pressure improved with results averaging 5.5 mmHg for the diastolic reading and 7.5 mmHg for the systolic.

The effect of a lower carb approach on the whole practice and in the community.

My psychologist wife, Jen, had experience running groups of patients with chronic diseases. She pointed out that, given the level of interest, it would be more efficient, and more fun, to help people in groups of 20. We set up evening sessions, so that working people could attend, particularly encouraging partners and family members to come along. During these sessions, we shared information about just how 'sugary' carbs really were. We educated patients about nutrition, healthy fats and essential fat soluble vitamins. We also ran cookery demonstrations. Perhaps the greatest value, however, came from the group dynamic, whereby patients helped each other. Some people went on to become 'patient experts': it is particularly encouraging and motivational to meet someone you can identify with, who has already sorted themselves out.

While this was going on, more of the intrigued practice staff tried the diet and liked it. This meant that, after a few months, we had eight staff and doctors 'low carbing'. They, as well as our 'patient experts', spread the word through the community, so the benefits began to show well beyond the study group.

I think that it is important to 'practise as I preach'. This has given me better insights into problems, which can occur in the early days. In the interests of balance and safety, here are a few things to look out for, which I have noticed with lower-carbohydrate regimes & T2DM:

- Muscle cramps can be experienced. This is likely due to a potassium/sodium short-term imbalance as people tend to lose sodium and so may need extra salt in the early days of going low-carb;

- Hypotension (low blood pressure) can be experienced, particularly in those on blood pressure lowering medications who lose a significant amount of weight. The good news is that the blood pressure medication may need to be reduced, or stopped altogether. Do work closely with your GP if you cut back on carbohydrate intake dramatically and take blood pressure medications;

- Hypoglycemia (low blood glucose) can be experienced, usually only for people on diabetic medication. This may need to be reviewed with your GP/consultant.

For any doctors reading this, blood glucose control should improve with patients reducing their carbohydrate intake. Be aware that, although in my experience, dietary sources of sugar are the commonest immediate cause of diabetes, other things like stress and medications may be important. And finally, if you see a patient losing weight, while HbA1c is rising, it may be pertinent to consider the (very rare) possibility of carcinoma pancreas and arrange a scan to examine this further.

By practising what I preach, not only do I have better insights into what patients are going through, I find that the patients trust me more. I'm not handing them a diet sheet, which I haven't personally tried. As for my own benefit? It's been immense. I feel younger. I have more energy. I need less sleep. I hardly ever need painkillers and I can run a 52 minute 10K, on low carbohydrate intake, aged 58.

The results of offering the approach at a practice level over 3 years, involving 850 people with diabetes or pre-diabetes have been as follows:

- Overall practice markers for diabetes control have improved: Nationally the English primary-care (Quality and Outcome Framework) marker of successful diabetic control is a HbA1c of

175

≤59 mmol/mol. Previously, 59.6% of our patients met this target, now 65.4% of patients do so, an improvement of 5.8% (absolute difference). This compares with an average achievement for England of 60.4%;

- Savings on insulin and drugs for diabetes: Our practice spends approximately £40,000 less per year than is average for the area. In part, this is because we now routinely give newly diagnosed people with diabetes the option of a dietary trial *before* starting lifelong medication. Not a single patient has opted for the drug option in three years.

A pleasant bonus for patients was that they noticed shrinking waistlines. In our initial pilot study, the average waist circumference reduced by 14 cms. The World Health Organization is concerned about so-called *Central Obesity*. In *Obesity: Preventing and Managing the Global Epidemic. Report of a WHO consultation* (2000), it was reported that the risk of metabolic complications was substantially increased: in men with a waist measurement greater than 102 cm; and in women with a waist measurement greater than 88 cm. Hence, this reduction in belly size could be clinically important. Insulin has been termed 'fat fertiliser' and it is possible that a lower carb diet helps improve central obesity via a reduction in insulin production.

Having reviewed these results, although stress, lack of exercise and other factors like medication (statins, steroids, diuretics) are possible causes of diabetes, I have come to the conclusion that, for most people with T2DM, dietary sources of glucose are the most likely and potentially remediable factors worth pursuing. This is why I have concentrated so much of my energy on the best way to help my patients to reduce dietary sugars and refined carbohydrates.

Where's the sugar?

I start conversations with my patients by asking *Where do you think the sugar is in your diet?* This at least gets us thinking about dietary sources of sugar. Some immediately mention sugar in hot drinks, or sweets, cakes and chocolate bars, but a significant number are mystified as they have "already cut most of the sugar out of their diet."

This leads me to wonder where the hidden sugars are in that patient's diet. To discover this, I find 'The breakfast question' invaluable. Ask a patient what they have for breakfast and, so often the answers include toast, breakfast biscuits, cereals, bananas or fruit juice. All of which, the general public do not associate with high-glycaemic index sources of large amounts of dietary glucose. But how sugary are these more modern breakfast foods compared to eggs for instance? For this we need to go back to the glycemic index.

There is a lot of published research on the ability of both the glycaemic index (GI already mentioned) and the associated glycaemic load (GL) to help predict the effect on blood glucose of the various carbohydrates in our foods against a standard of pure glucose. We know, for example, that the carbohydrate in boiled rice is far more 'sugary' than an equivalent amount of the carbohydrate from, say, boiled spaghetti. In practice we found that both clinicians and patients lacked experience with glucose and struggled to use it as a reference point. So, with help from Dr Geoff Livesey, a well-known carbohydrate expert, I experimented with a re-interpretation of the data, but this time using the far more familiar concept of a teaspoon of sugar (4 g of sugar). Figure 1 shows the conversion of glucose in foods into teaspoons of sugar. This figure was published in the Journal of Insulin Resistance.[10]

FIGURE 1

Food Item	Glycaemic index	Serve size g	How does each food affect blood glucose compared with one 4g teaspoon of table sugar?
Basmati rice	69	150	10.1
Potato, white, boiled	96	150	9.1
French Fries baked	64	150	7.5
Spaghetti White boiled	39	180	6.6
Sweet corn boiled	60	80	4.0
Frozen peas, boiled	51	80	1.3
Banana	62	120	5.7
Apple	39	120	2.3
Wholemeal Small slice	74	30	3.0
Broccoli	54	80	0.2
Eggs	60	0	

Other foods in the very low glycaemic range would be chicken, oily fish, almonds, mushrooms, cheese

177

Returning to the question of 'where is the sugar in your diet?' we can use our 'teaspoons of table sugar equivalent' system to help inform dietary choices. So many people think that naturally occurring sugars are 'healthy.' However, for someone with diabetes, looking at figure 2, we can see that a banana, some raisins or apple juice are the glycaemic equivalent of a surprisingly large number of teaspoons of sugar. Foods with added sugar are a second source of glucose. This system allows patients to compare digestive biscuits with malt loaf or other foods. A third and final source of glucose is starchy non-sweet food, which is digested (broken down) into glucose. Of the three sources, I find that this one is the most often forgotten. Many people are startled to see the teaspoon of sugar equivalents of brown bread, rice or a baked potato. (Although those readers with a blood glucose meter may not be so surprised!).*

FIGURE 2

Three different sources of sugars that make up our total dietary 'sugar burden'; shown as 4g teaspoon of table sugar equivalents*		
1 Naturally occurring sugars	2 Foods with added sugars	3 Foods digested down into sugars
Banana 4.9 teaspoons/100g	Coco Pops®, average 24.4teaspoons/100g	Brown bread 10.8 teaspoons/100g
Honey 17.6 teaspoons/100g	Fanta orange 3.4 teaspoons/100ml	Boiled spaghetti 3.7 teaspoons/100g
Skimmed Milk 0.9 teaspoons/100ml	Digestive biscuits 8.8 teaspoons/100g	French fries 5.1 teaspoons/100g
Raisins 17.1 teaspoons/100g	Malt loaf 14.7 teaspoons/100g	Basmati rice 6.8 teaspoons/100g
Apple juice 4.3 teaspoons/100ml	Rasberry yoghurt 2.4 teaspoons/100g	Baked potato 6.3 teaspoons/100g

*As each food would effect blood glucose, from the International tables of glycaemic index and glycaemic load (Atkinson, Foster-Powell et al. 2008) as per the calculations in a paper published by The Journal of Insulin Resistance 'It's the glycaemic response to, not the carbohydrate content of food that matters in diabetes and obesity: The glycaemic index revisited.' D J Unwin et al.

Just looking again at my breakfast question, we can work out the equivalents:

---

* A flaw in my table sugar equivalent system is that in fact table sugar is a mixture of the sugar in question, glucose and also fructose, which has some separate health concerns of its own. But this being said, in practice I have found as a system it really helps people with diabetes to a better understanding of the blood glucose consequences of their dietary choices.

A breakfast of 30 g CocoPops (8 teasp), plus milk (125 ml) (1 teasp), plus just one small slice of brown toast (3 teasp) with 200 ml apple juice (8-9 teasp) is equivalent to a surprising twenty (20) 4 g spoons of sugar in terms of the effect on blood glucose over 2 hours. Even substituting the decadent CocoPops with a spartan 30 g of Branflakes still leaves our conventional breakfast at an equivalent of 16 spoonfuls of table sugar. Compare this to a three egg cheese omelette, which will struggle to be the equivalent of even just one or two spoonfuls of sugar (Figure 3). Looking at this information set out in figure 3, it can easily be seen why the UK 2015 NICE guidelines for T2DM advise low-glycaemic index sources of carbohydrate in the diet.

FIGURE 3

Two very different breakfasts: 1- cereals, toast, fruit juice. 2 three egg cheese & mushroom omelette with tomato, coffee. How might each breakfast effect blood glucose ?*			
food item		Serving size in g/ml	How does each food affect blood glucose compared with one 4g teaspoon of table sugar?
Bran flakes	Breakfast 1	30	3.7
milk	Breakfast 1	125	1 Total for breakfast 1, 16.3 teaspoons
Brown toast, 1 slice	Breakfast 1	30	3
Pure Apple juice	Breakfast 1	200	8.6
Eggs, (little carb)	Breakfast 2	90	<0.1
Mushrooms	Breakfast 2	30	0.1
Cheese,(little carb)	Breakfast 2	25	<0.1 Total for breakfast 2, <1 teaspoon
Tomato	Breakfast 2	50	0.1
Coffee with milk	Breakfast 2	25ml milk	0.2
Possibly useful information for someone with type 2 diabetes making dietary choices			

*As per calculations derived from the glycaemic index, to be found in: It's the glycaemic response to, not the carbohydrate content of food that matters in diabetes and obesity Journal of Insulin Resistance 2016. Unwin et al

"He is the best physician who is the most ingenious inspirer of hope." Samuel Taylor Coleridge about 1810

I have mentioned my wife, Jen already. She is a consultant health psychologist who has spent many years looking into the role of hope in chronic conditions. Psychologists are experts at changing behaviour and sugar consumption has many psychological aspects, which need combating. Working alongside a psychologist with this programme made me realise the mistake I had been making over the years. I had played too much on fear and not enough on hope. Too much of my language with patients was 'threatening' and involved dire warnings around diabetes.

Working together, our practice discovered how it is far better to motivate and inspire people, than to worry and scare them. We worked to understand what our patients' goals were – for their health and weight. Some wanted to avoid medication; most people want to look and feel younger. For others, the simple, practical goal of "breathing better" was top of the list. We then worked with people to help them to understand what a significant difference diet could make with these health and weight goals – if the person chose to take this option. Unsurprisingly, they were keen to try something that could help them to achieve their goals.

In this way, reducing dietary glucose was placed into an appropriate psychological setting. I also found that regular 'medical result' feedback greatly encouraged commitment, as part of ongoing support. Most doctors are reluctant to measure glycosylated haemoglobin (HbA1c) more frequently than every three to six months. I think that this is a shame as significant improvements can be seen after only six weeks, which can be a great boost to confidence. The scales and one's favourite jeans, of course, are the patient's own measure of success. Some patients may curse us for the cost of new wardrobes, but lives have been transformed because an old dog learned some new tricks.

Dr David Unwin

@lowcarbGP

Case Study: Lindy

Lindy was devastated to learn that she had Type 2 Diabetes. Her GP's (General Practitioner) advice was daily metformin and a high-carb diet. But Lindy did her own research, and found a different solution. Less than a year on, Lindy says that she is fitter, healthier, and the box of metformin has remained unopened.

For many years I had a hectic life working as a Personal Assistant in blue chip global companies, but now I've reached 52, my husband and I have moved to the lovely Scottish Highlands to open a Bed & Breakfast business.

Looking back, I was always healthy and active. I walked, rode horses and ate healthily, both as a child, and then as an adult in Cyprus. Food was very healthy there – always fresh, with emphasis on meats, salads and very little carbs. I was the healthiest and fittest I have ever been.

A new relationship brought me to Holland, where riding took a back seat to a high-carb diet and full-time stressful job. As we returned

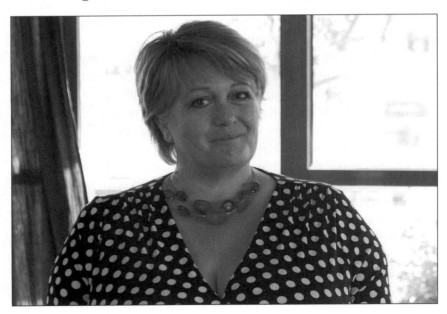

back to the UK in 2012, I was well aware that I would be leaving Holland around 40 kg heavier than when I'd arrived.

Fast-forward to 2016: I was feeling horrible, bloated, tired, crabby, achy and my eyesight was starting to fail.

Concerned at the rapid worsening of my eyesight, my optician sent me to the GP for tests, and that's when my world collapsed.

My HbA1c had come back at 118 mmol/mol or 17.7 mmol/L – I was an off-the-scale Type 2 diabetic! My blood pressure was also concerning and they were also muttering about high cholesterol at 7.7 mmol/L.

My ears still ringing to phrases like "diabetic for life... insulin is inevitable... amputation is a very real possibility", I left the surgery with a three-month supply of metformin (2000 mg/day), advice to eat a high-carb diet, and a return appointment date for three months.

I hit the absolute deck for about two days. I was very scared, very ashamed, and convinced that I was going to die.

Then my inner control-freak kicked in.

I'd read Zoë Harcombe's book a few years previously, but now it was time to act on it. I researched all her articles on Diabetes – along with the Diet Doctor, Jason Fung and others – and decided that I was going to attack this with a lifestyle change for three months, then review progress.

I convinced my husband that if the results were positive, then the drugs would remain unopened. (To be honest, I also wanted to do the lifestyle change and did not want any argument that it was the tablets that had done the work and not me).

I bought myself a blood glucose meter – thanks to my hubby for helping me with my fear of needles – and started to take readings on waking, before each meal and two hours after each meal.

I stuck to a LCHF diet ensuring that I did not go over 20 grams of carbs a day and slowly started to build up a list of meals that I knew I could eat with no or little effect on my blood glucose.

Food was certainly not boring: chicken roasted in herby goose fat with salad and feta cheese; deconstructed burgers with cheese, salad, gherkins and mayo; roasted duck legs with garlic beans; slow roasted lamb with salad and feta and olives.

I rediscovered my love of exercising, and got back into the swing of regular morning and evening dog walks.

And what was the result? Guess what: my readings were coming down, as were my weekly blood sugar averages... and the weight was flying off too. In fact, within twelve weeks, I had lost the three stone that I'd gained in Holland!

I got the official results from my GP when I returned for my three-month check-up.

My HbA1c was down from 118 to 44 mmol/mol, which is in low pre-diabetic ranges, and this gave me an average blood glucose reading of 7.3 mmol/L (it had been 17.7).

My blood pressure was normal at 130/80, and my cholesterol levels had dropped from 7.7 to 5.9 mmol/L.

I'd also lost 24 kg, four dress sizes, and three bra sizes!

All of this was achieved with no medication, lots of natural good food, and certainly not shirking away from fat.

My GP was pleased that my results had dramatically improved, but he showed no interest in how I had done it. Yet I took great delight in handing back his unopened pack of metformin.

Eight months on and things are good on my low-carb lifestyle. My bloods are stable, I sleep better, wake up feeling rested, have more energy, and seem happier all round.

If you had asked me a year ago, I would have said weight-loss was the main driver, the most important thing, but now I see it as a happy by-product of feeling so well, fit and healthy.

In fact, I have no idea what I weigh, only that I've dropped another dress size and feel great in my clothes.

One last thing: I agreed to share my story in this book because I was invited to share my advice to those readers who are in the position I was this time last year.

I too was blaming myself. I too was in a panic and scared about amputations and blindness and a lifetime of medication to stave it off.

So my advice to you is simple: take control of your own health.

Rather than accepting the view of your GP or Health Care Professional as sacrosanct, do your own research and ask questions and follow your own judgement. It is YOUR life after all.

I, for one, have no doubts that had I blindly followed the advice given to me by my practice nurse this time last year, I'd be sat here today looking at my latest high HbA1c results; full of worry and self-blame. I'd be eagerly accepting an increasing cocktail of meds as the only option.

I certainly wouldn't be enjoying life more than ever; and never would have felt the anger, sadness, and delight I am feeling at this keyboard now.

The big issues

Chapter Eleven

Why do we eat so much carbohydrate?

by Dr Zoë Harcombe, Ph.D

There's a really short answer to this question and there's an answer that took me three to four years to bottom out because it was the subject of my Ph.D. My Ph.D was entitled: "An examination of the randomised controlled trial and epidemiological evidence for the introduction of dietary fat recommendations in 1977 and 1983: A Systematic Review and Meta-Analysis." What a mouthful! What that means is that I looked at the dietary fat recommendations, which were introduced in 1977 in the US and 1983 in the UK and I looked at the evidence for those guidelines. I looked at the evidence in four parts: what was the randomised controlled trial (RCT) evidence at the time the guidelines were introduced?; what RCT evidence would be available today if the guideline committee were meeting?; what was the epidemiological evidence at the time the guidelines were introduced?; what epidemiological evidence would be available today if the guideline committee were meeting?

RCT evidence is of higher value than epidemiological evidence. The way in which research is supposed to work is that epidemiological observation should identify an association between two things and then an RCT should be conducted to test if that observation is causal. e.g. it may be observed that a population (let's call them chimney sweeps) develop scrotal cancer and a comparator population (not chimney sweeps) didn't develop scrotal cancer. Researchers should then do a trial where they randomly allocated, say 100 people to become chimney sweeps and 100 people to not become chimney sweeps (keeping everything else the same between the 200 people, as far as possible) and then study the people for long enough to see if there is a significant difference in incidence of scrotal cancer.

I use this example, because this is one of the populations (chimney sweeps) and conditions (scrotal cancer), which prompted Bradford

Hill to develop the first of what became known as "The Bradford Hill criteria"[1] – the strength of the association. Hill observed that deaths of chimney sweeps from scrotal cancer were "some 200 times" that of workers who were not chimney sweeps. That's as strong as it gets. Few people could see the strength of that relationship and fail to conclude that being a chimney sweep *causes* scrotal cancer. In this case, an RCT would *not* be necessary, but there have been no such overwhelming and irrefutable results in the field of nutrition – quite the contrary.

The short answer to the title of this chapter is as follows. There are only three things that we eat: carbohydrate, protein and fat (macronutrients). Protein tends to stay fairly constant (at 15-20% of total calorie intake) and so the macronutrients that vary are carbohydrate and fat. We eat so much carbohydrate because we demonised fat. The dietary fat guidelines set were that we should consume no more than 30% of our calorie intake in the form of total fat and no more than 10% in the form of saturated fat. With protein at, let's say, 15% – as soon as an upper limit is set on fat of 30%, the remainder necessarily must come from carbohydrate – 55%. The US dietary guideline literature spelled this out by recommending that 55-60% of the US diet should come from carbohydrate.

That's the short answer. The really interesting question is – why did we demonise fat? Seat belts on? Let's go...

(The following is the final chapter of my Ph.D, adjusted only to remove references to other chapters. It has been published as a peer reviewed paper.[2])

An examination of the randomised controlled trial and epidemiological evidence for the introduction of dietary fat recommendations in 1977 and 1983: A Systematic Review and Meta-Analysis.

The final chapter of this Ph.D

by Dr Zoë Harcombe

"The urgency of finding means of prevention is sharpest for men in middle age for it is in that group that the social cost of CHD is greatest... Starting with men aged 40 through 59, the follow-up would show CHD causing close to 40% of all deaths in five years. It is understandable, then, that most work on the epidemiology of CHD begins with men of those ages."

Ancel Keys (p. I-1)[3].

Introduction

The first part of the diet-heart hypothesis, that serum cholesterol was related to coronary heart disease (CHD), originated from the work of Russian pathologists in the early twentieth century. Having observed fatty deposits in arteries during post mortems, a number of researchers sought to understand if dietary cholesterol determined serum cholesterol[4-12]. The summary of findings from the original animal studies was that: rabbits (herbivores) fed animal foods developed fatty deposits/changes in the aortas; rats (omnivores) fed animal foods produced no observable changes in the aortas; and rabbits fed cholesterol in plant food showed no arterial damage.

In the 1950s, Keys undertook several experiments with human subjects and concluded "that the cholesterol content, per se, of all natural diets has *no* significant effect on either the serum cholesterol level or the development of atherosclerosis in man" (p. 182)[13].

In the early 1950s, literature referred to animal and vegetable fat and not the degree of saturation of fat[14-16]. Interventions with vegetable fat were extrapolated to conclusions about animal fat, without animal fat having been tested[15, 16].

The first references to saturated and unsaturated fats occurred later in the decade[17]. Keys' earliest findings were that there was

189

no relationship between the saturation of fats and their effects in producing hypercoagulability of the blood after they were eaten[17].

The second part of the diet-heart hypothesis, that dietary fat and serum cholesterol were related, followed observational studies of men in Minnesota, Naples, Slough and Madrid. Keys concluded that the total fat content of the diet (as a proportion of calories) exerted a powerful influence on the serum cholesterol level in man[18]. Age appeared to be a confounder, with cholesterol rising to the age of 50-55 in Minnesotan and Slough men and rich men in Madrid. Neapolitan men and poor men in Madrid demonstrated stable and falling cholesterol levels respectively between the ages of 40 and 50; rising before these ages.

The third part of the diet-heart hypothesis, that dietary fat and CHD were related, was first presented with the graph of deaths from heart disease and calories from total fat in men aged 55-59, for six countries, from the Mount Sinai presentation of 1953[19]. The response of Yerushalmy and Hilleboe demonstrated that data were available for 22 countries[20].

Keys concluded that no other variable, besides the fat calories in the diet, showed anything like such a consistent relationship to the mortality rate from CHD[13].

The first statement of the diet-heart hypothesis, with the three component parts, appears to have been made in a 1955 publication, which explored the relationship between dietary fat, serum cholesterol and CHD in different ethnic groups in Cape Town[21]. This paper confirmed that total fat intake and animal fat intake were the subjects of examination. Saturated fat was not mentioned.

In 1957, Keys published another summary paper on "Diet and the epidemiology of coronary heart disease"[22]. Keys' position on fat, cholesterol and heart disease became more certain. He described the American diet as dominated by "innumerable fat-loading meals", the results of which were "hypercholesteremia, which promotes atherosclerosis". Keys differentiated that food fats were not identical in promoting hypercholesteremia, but those most prevalent in fatty diets were more powerful in this direction than food oils that had an opposing effect. As a final complication, Keys noted that different fats had differing effects on serum cholesterol and blood coagulation (p. 1912)[22].

This was the context for the start of The Seven Countries Study in 1956-1958. The Seven Countries Study concluded that there was no relationship with total fat and CHD, but that there was a strong correlation between saturated fat intake and CHD in one of seven countries when compared with saturated fat intake and CHD in others of seven countries[3].

In ideal research circumstances, epidemiological evidence would have established clear and consistent associations and then well designed randomised controlled trials (RCTs) would have followed epidemiological findings and set out to test associations found. This did not happen with the development of the diet-heart hypothesis. Possibly the sense of urgency took over. The epidemiology and RCTs were running in parallel from the 1950s onwards.

The focus on men, and men who had already had a heart attack in the case of the RCTs, was understandable in the context of the Keys' quotation at the top of p. 189. This focus, however, lacked generalisability for the population as a whole.

Results

The findings

Public health advice for all citizens should be informed by conclusive, consistent, evidence from numerous robust studies, of an appropriate representative group of such citizens (large enough, long enough, studies of healthy men and women of all ages). This did not happen before the guidelines were set. It has not happened since and it is unlikely to happen in the future, not least with cost, ethical and confounding variable complications, such as the prevalence of medication. There are two issues with the evidence examined in this thesis:

1) The conclusions of the evidence:

The evidence available to the dietary committees at the time the guidelines were introduced did not support the recommendations made. A systematic review and meta-analysis of RCTs available in 1977/1983, where a dietary fat intervention had been made, revealed identical all-cause mortality (30% in intervention and control

191

groups) and no statistically significant difference in deaths from CHD.[23] A systematic review of prospective cohort studies available in 1977/1983 found one study offering support for saturated, but not total fat, to be a subject for further examination and five studies with no significant findings in relation to total, or saturated, dietary fat.[24]

The evidence currently available offers no additional support. A systematic review and meta-analysis of dietary fat RCTs currently available, where a dietary fat intervention had been made, found no statistically significant difference in all-cause mortality or deaths from CHD.[25] A systematic review and meta-analysis of prospective cohort studies currently available found no statistically significant results to implicate total or saturated fat in CHD mortality.[26]

With one exception, the specific guidelines of 30% total fat and 10% saturated fat have not been tested. The STARS[27] was the only study to examine targets approximating to those set by dietary guidelines, with a total fat consumption of 27% and an 8-10% saturated fat intake. The DART[28] tested a 30% total fat diet, although this was not a controlled variable, as the intervention also tried to achieve a 1:1 polyunsaturated to saturated fat ratio. Two RCTs studied an approximate 20% fat diet[29, 30]. Two reviewed the consequence of a 10% saturated fat diet, without the total fat dietary guideline restriction[31, 32]. The prospective cohort studies examined grams of fat intake for those who died from CHD vs. those who didn't, or fat intake as a percentage of calories, sometimes in absolute amounts, sometimes comparing lowest and highest tertiles, quartiles or quintiles. They did not examine populations for outcomes related to the two dietary fat guidelines. This is not a criticism of the studies. Public health policy should follow evidence, not the other way round.

One RCT claimed that its findings supported the use of a lipid-lowering diet in men with CHD[27]. Three prospective cohort studies reported strong evidence for an association between dietary fat and CHD: The Seven Countries Study found an association with saturated fat[33]; Boniface and Tefft[34] found an association with both total and saturated fat, but for men only, not women; Xu *et al* found associations for total fat, saturated fatty acid and monounsaturated fatty acid intake in American Indians aged 47-59 years, but not older[35].

All other RCTs and prospective cohort studies reported no significant findings for total or saturated dietary fat. Four RCTs issued cautions about the safety and/or efficacy of their interventions[29, 31, 36, 37]. Rose *et al* reported that corn oil was most unlikely to be beneficial, and was possibly harmful[36]. The Research Committee Low-fat Diet concluded that a low-fat diet has no place in the treatment of myocardial infarction[29]. Dayton *et al* noted the absence of any benefit for longevity and expressed concern about toxicity of the intervention[37]. Woodhill *et al* reported that survival was significantly better in the control than the diet group[31].

Regarding the serum cholesterol part of the diet-heart hypothesis, the RCTs at the time and currently available collectively reported greater reductions in mean serum cholesterol levels in the intervention groups, but this did not result in a reduction in deaths, from CHD or all-causes. These findings raise questions about the mechanism of cholesterol lowering medications, such as statins. It has been assumed that statins lower cholesterol and lowering cholesterol lowers death rates. There may be another mechanism by which statins have an effect, independent of cholesterol. Caution should be adopted in using cholesterol as a surrogate end-point: the new Proprotein convertase subtilisin/kexin type 9 inhibitors (PCSK9) are being launched with surrogate end-point evidence alone, without evidence for CHD mortality[38].

Plant sterols offer a plausible explanation for dietary interventions lowering cholesterol, but not mortality. Plant sterols is the collective term for free and esterified phytosterols and phytostanols, regardless of biological source. Phytosterols are cholesterol-like molecules found in all plant foods, with the highest concentrations occurring in vegetable oils. They are absorbed only in trace amounts, but inhibit the absorption of intestinal cholesterol[39]. The most commonly occurring phytosterols in the human diet are β-sitosterol, campesterol and stigmasterol, which account for approximately 65%, 30% and 3% of diet contents respectively[40]. The ability of phytosterols to inhibit the absorption of cholesterol was first established in 1953[41]. However, there is no evidence that plant sterols reduce the risk of CHD and much evidence that they are detrimental[42].

2) The quality of the evidence:

Even if the evidence from prospective cohort studies and RCTs had been overwhelming, the limitations of the studies were so great that the evidence could not be relied upon. Only one RCT was a primary study of both men and women[32]. Only one prospective cohort study, with evidence for CHD mortality, examined both men and women, free from CHD at the baseline[43]. All prospective cohort studies suffered the limitations of dietary questionnaires[44-49]. Other limitations of each study have been documented in the published papers[23-26].

The Seven Countries Study

The strongest evidence presented, among 10 RCTs and 13 prospective cohort studies, came from The Seven Countries Study[33]. Keys noted in the introduction to The Seven Countries Study publication that association did not mean causation, but the strength of conclusions did not adopt this caution. The conclusions of this study defined the diet-heart hypothesis as the tripartite association of saturated fat, serum cholesterol levels and CHD; the impact of dietary cholesterol and total dietary fat having been rejected[33].

The correlations established by The Seven Countries Study were strong. The correlation between median serum cholesterol level and CHD deaths and infarctions (data for CHD deaths alone were not presented) per 100 people was $r = 0.76$ ($p<0.05$). The correlation between CHD deaths and infarctions and saturated fat as a percentage of calories was $r = 0.84$ ($p<0.05$)[50]. However, these correlations were for countries vs. each other, not for people in one country who died from CHD vs. those in the same country who didn't.

The confounders were significant, including, but not limited to: geography; lifestyle; Gross Domestic Product; climate; politics; other aspects of national diet; national health provision etc. When asked about the value of Keys' work, a contemporary of the time, Professor Peter Elwood, described inter country studies as "the lowest form of evidence"[51].

The Seven Countries Study suffered from further limitations with the pre-selection of countries known to be associated; an average of 3.4% of men sampled for dietary information; and the inclusion of men with pre-existing CHD, with the finding that the CHD death rate within 5 years was 20.9% for secondary males and 1.0% for primary males.

Without these limitations, the strong correlations established by The Seven Countries Study were not unique. Equally strong correlations had been established with animal protein, with Gross Domestic Product suggested as the confounder[20]; television sets and vehicle licenses[52]; and the strongest correlation of all was established with latitude in this thesis.

A definitive assessment of the strength of associations found in research was proposed by Bradford Hill with his nine criteria[1]. In 2009, Mente *et al* reviewed RCTs and prospective cohort studies against these criteria for numerous foods and nutrients. They concluded: "**Insufficient evidence** of association is present for intake of ... saturated and polyunsaturated fatty acids; total fat; linolenic acid; meat; eggs and milk" (p. 659)[53].

Although The Seven Countries Study was not referenced by the US committee February publication[54], it was referenced by the UK committee[55] and Keys and his research was referenced 40 times in the 869 supplemental pages to the dietary guidelines[56]. The fact that Keys had appeared on the front cover of Time Magazine attested to the regard with which he was held[57]. There can be little doubt that The Seven Countries Study had a significant impact on the introduction of dietary fat guidelines.

Other meta-analyses

A number of meta-analyses of RCTs have been undertaken by other authors[58-61]. A meta-analysis of prospective cohort studies has been undertaken by other authors[62]. Two additional meta-analyses reviewed both RCTs and prospective cohort studies[63, 64]. Skeaff and Miller sought to summarise the evidence from cohort studies and RCTs of the relation between dietary fat and risk of CHD. Their conclusion was "Intake of total fat was not significantly associated with CHD mortality. Intake of total fat was also unrelated to CHD events" (p. 175)[63]. Chowdhury *et al* set out to summarise evidence between fatty acids and coronary disease. Their review examined saturated, monounsaturated, polyunsaturated and trans fats, while also reviewing individual chain length fatty acids, palmitic (C16:0) and margaric (C17:0) as examples. The conclusion was "Current evidence does not clearly support cardiovascular guidelines that encourage high consumption of polyunsaturated fatty acids and low consumption of total saturated fats" (p. 398)[64].

Table 7.1 summarises the findings from other meta-analyses of RCTs and/or prospective cohort studies. Table 7.2 reports their objectives and inclusion criteria. There were 39 reports of risk ratios from meta-analysis with 95% confidence intervals. Of these, 4 reported significant findings; 35 reported no significant findings. One of the significant findings related to trans fats, not total or saturated fat. It found that trans fat intake was positively associated with coronary disease[64]. Another of the significant findings came from the study of the impact of replacing saturated fat with polyunsaturated fat[60], which was criticised[65] for excluding two studies that would have moderated this conclusion[31, 36] and including a favourable, but non-randomised cross-over, trial excluded by all other meta-analyses[66, 67].

The other two significant findings were related to CVD events and not mortality[59, 61]. In 2011, including RCTs with a minimum of 6 months duration, Hooper *et al* found 1 significant result and 11 non-significant results. The one significant result was that, when all RCTs were examined together, the risk ratio (RR) for CVD events from meta-analysis was 0.86 (95% CI 0.77 to 0.96). In 2015, including RCTs with a minimum of 24 months duration, Hooper *et al* found one significant result and seven non-significant results. The one significant result was, when a reduction in saturated fat was examined, the risk ratio (RR) for CVD events from meta-analysis was 0.83 (95% CI 0.72 to 0.96).

As a result of this 2015 review, Hooper *et al* suggested that there may be a small reduction in cardiovascular risk with reduction of saturated fat intake[61]. It was further suggested that replacing the energy from saturated fat with polyunsaturated fat "appears to be a useful strategy, and replacement with carbohydrate appears less useful" (p. 2)[61] and replacement with monounsaturated fat unclear. Of the 11 interventions contributing to this conclusion, only 1 documented both saturated fat reduction and reported that this was mainly replaced with polyunsaturated fat[37].

The Hooper meta-analyses of 2011 and 2015 included four small studies (646 people in total), not included in any other meta-analysis, which were primarily studies of: diabetes[68]; skin cancer[69]; hypercholesterolemia[70]; and glucose intolerance[71], but for which Hooper *et al* obtained CVD event information. The most recent review[61] included no study of healthy people of both genders. The

196

one primary, both-sex RCT available was excluded by Hooper *et al*, for not meeting the 24 month duration criteria[32]. The one significant finding of small benefit for CVD events, among numerous insignificant findings, thus also lacked generalisability.

Dietary fat guidelines were introduced with the ambition of reducing deaths from CHD. No meta-analysis of RCTs and/or prospective cohort studies has found any significant difference for dietary fat interventions and all-cause mortality or deaths from CHD, or associations with dietary fat and CHD mortality[23, 58-64].

Discussion

Have there been consequences?

Both the US and UK documents acknowledged that the evidence was not conclusive. The UK publication referred to "a strong consensus of opinion" (p. 24)[55]. Hegsted's introduction to the Dietary Goals for The United States noted "there will undoubtedly be many people who will say we have not proven our point" (p. 3)[54].

Hegsted continued by asking "What are the risks associated with eating less meat, less fat, less saturated fat, less cholesterol, less sugar, less salt, and more fruits, vegetables, unsaturated fat and cereal products – especially whole grain cereals. There are none that can be identified" (p. 8)[54].

Senators Percy, Schweiker and Zorinsky wrote a foreword for the second edition of the guidelines noting the "lack of consensus among nutritional scientists and other health professionals" (p. vii). They recommended that it be stated in bold print on the Goals and Food Selection pages "that the value of dietary change remains controversial and that science cannot at this time insure (sic) that an altered diet will improve protection from certain killer diseases such as heart disease and cancer" (p. ix)[72].

The second edition of the US dietary goals was published at the end of 1977[72]. In between the first edition[54] and the second, many witnesses appeared before the committee. Deliberations were reflected in a number of comments from the second edition of the guidelines: "Some witnesses have claimed that physical harm could result from the diet modifications recommended in this report...

197

However, after further review, the Select Committee still finds that no physical or mental harm could result from the dietary guidelines recommended for the general public"(p. xxxiii)[72]. The view was, therefore, that even if benefit were unproven, no harm could be done.

There are three macronutrients: carbohydrate; protein and fat. Protein is found in all foods except pure fats (oils and lard) and sucrose[73]. The proportion of protein in a natural diet thus tends to remain constant at approximately 15-20% of energy intake. If fat intake is reduced, as a proportion of energy intake, carbohydrate concomitantly rises. The consequences of increasing carbohydrate content in human diets had not been investigated before the dietary fat guidelines were introduced.

Until the introduction of dietary guidelines in 1977, the view of Tanner, from The Practice of Medicine, prevailed "Farinaceous and vegetable foods are fattening, and saccharine matters are especially so" (p. 213)[74]. In 1960, 13.3% of United States (US) adults were obese; 44.8% were overweight. By 2007, 34.7% of US adults were obese; 67.7% were overweight[75]. In the UK, in 1972, 2.7% of men and 2.7% of women were obese and 23.0% of men and 13.9% of women were overweight. By 1999, obesity rates had risen to 22.6% of men and 25.8% of women, while 49.2% of men and 36.3% of women were overweight[76]. (Health was devolved in the UK in 1999 to the regions of England, Northern Ireland, Scotland and Wales and thus UK statistics terminated).

The diabetes rate was 2.4% in 1976 in the US[77]. The introduction to the 2010 Dietary Guidelines for Americans reported that 24 million Americans, almost 11% of the adult population, were diabetic and 78 million Americans, 35% of adults were pre-diabetic[78]. This has recently been updated to 29 million diabetics and 86 million pre-diabetics[79]. A recent review in The Lancet, estimated that the lifetime risk for developing diabetes was 40.2% for American men and 39.6% for women[80]. There were 800,000 people with diabetes in the UK in 1980, from a population of 56 million – an incident rate of 1.42%[81]. The diabetes rate in the UK in 2015 was 6.1%[82]. The incident rate of diabetes, in both the US and the UK, has increased more than four fold since the dietary fat guidelines were introduced.

The association between the introduction of the dietary fat guidelines and concomitant increases in obesity and diabetes deserves examination. A number of recent reviews have suggested a causal connection: "The replacement of saturated fats in the diet with carbohydrates, especially sugars, has resulted in increased obesity and its associated health complications" (p. 294)[83]. In a BMJ Editorial, cardiologist, Dr Aseem Malhotra closed with the statement: "It is time to bust the myth of the role of saturated fat in heart disease and wind back the harms of dietary advice that has contributed to obesity" (p. 1)[84]. In 2014, Dr James DiNicolantino questioned current dietary guidelines. Having reviewed data trends for dietary fat and obesity in the US, he concluded: "These data provide a strong argument that the increase in the consumption of refined carbohydrates was the causative dietary factor for the diabetes and obesity epidemic in the USA" (p. 1)[85]. Following a Swedish systematic review of literature, an article was published in the BMJ entitled "Swedish health advisory body says too much carbohydrate, not fat, leads to obesity"[86]. Feinman *et al* analysed US dietary intake for the period 1974-2000 and concluded: "During the epidemics of obesity and Type 2 diabetes, caloric increases have been due almost entirely to increased carbohydrate" (p. 6)[87].

Dietary guidelines set to change?

The US dietary guidelines, originally issued in 1980, are re-issued every five years; 2015 being a dietary guidelines year of issue. The draft report for 2015, from the US dietary guidelines advisory committee (DGAC), was published in February 2015[88]. The recommendation to limit dietary cholesterol intake to 300 milligrams a day has prevailed in the US since 1977[54]. The DGAC stated that they will not bring forward this recommendation because available evidence shows no appreciable relationship between consumption of dietary cholesterol and serum cholesterol: "*Cholesterol is not a nutrient of concern for over consumption*" (p. 90)[88]. The UK did not introduce dietary cholesterol targets in the original guidelines[55, 89] and they have not been introduced since[90]. The Keys' research from the 1950s concluded that dietary cholesterol should never have been a nutrient of concern[13].

The DGAC advice demonstrated further movement away from the original dietary fat guidelines by containing no total fat recommendation and a change in the position on dietary fat and cardiovascular disease (CVD). The advisory report documented the findings of the

199

meta-analyses by Skeaff[63] (RCTs and prospective cohorts), Siri-Tarino[62] (prospective cohorts), Hooper[59] (RCTs) and Chowdhury[64] (RCTs and prospective cohorts) and concluded that reducing total fat does not lower CVD risk[88]. The saturated fat guideline was reiterated, however, with the recommendation to consume fewer than 10% of total calories from saturated fat per day[88].

There are consequences of maintaining the saturated fat guideline and not the total fat guideline. Consumption of one, or both, of the other natural fats, monounsaturated and polyunsaturated, may increase. The fat that is being promoted for higher intake is polyunsaturated fat[60, 61, 91-93]. Many authors have expressed concern about this recommendation[65, 85, 94-98].

It is important to differentiate between polyunsaturated fats. The DART provided early evidence for the benefit of omega-3 polyunsaturated fat, naturally abundant in fish[28]. The only significant finding from this RCT was that all-cause mortality was lower for those following the fish advice, which was to increase fatty fish intake to at least two portions (200-400 g) weekly. The relative risk for fish advice vs. no fish advice was 0.71 (0.54-0.92) ($p<0.05$) (table IV, p. 759)[28]. This significant finding was explored further by the research team, but not found to be replicated[99]. Omega-6 polyunsaturated fats have pro-inflammatory properties, which can be mitigated by omega-3 intake[100], but any dietary advice on polyunsaturated fats needs to be specific and evidence based.

The UK does not review dietary guidelines at regular intervals. The target for total fat remains 30% of daily total energy intake and 10% for saturated fat[90].

A way forward?

The 2010 Dietary Guidelines for Americans documented the sources of saturated fat in the American diet (fig. 3-4, p.26)[78]. Pizza, desserts, candy, potato chips, pasta, tortillas, burritos and tacos accounted for 32.6% of saturated fat consumed in the diets of US citizens aged 2 years and older. 9.3% of dietary saturated fat came from sausages, frankfurters, bacon, ribs and burgers. 12.8% came from chicken and mixed chicken dishes, beef and mixed beef dishes, and eggs and mixed egg dishes. A further 24.5% was unaccounted for and collated as "All other food categories"; likely including, if not predominantly being, processed foods. The natural foods listed were cheese, milk, butter, nuts and seeds which collectively accounted for 20.8% of saturated fat intake. It would have been ideal for unprocessed chicken, beef and eggs to have been separated from processed meals containing these ingredients. The diagram presented in the Dietary Guidelines is clear nonetheless. Processed foods account for the majority of saturated fat intake in the diets of Americans.

The UK classification is similar. The Family Food Survey (table 2.4, p. 18) documented sources of saturated fat in the UK diet[101]. Bread, cakes, buns, pastries, biscuits, cereals, confectionery and other processed foods accounted for 33% of saturated fat intake. Milk, cream and cheese accounted for 24% of dietary saturated fat. Processed meat accounted for 16% of saturated fat intake, while unprocessed (carcass) meat was 5%, fish 1% and eggs 1% of saturated fat intake. Fats and oils made up the remaining 19% (99% due to rounding errors). As with the US, processed food accounted for the majority of the saturated fat intake of the UK.

There is opportunity for strong agreement among health professionals. If the public health message were revised to advise citizens to eat natural food and not processed food, saturated fat intake would fall accordingly although the health benefit would likely be the concomitant reduction in sucrose, trans fats and other processed ingredients deleterious to human health. Human beings evolved to eat foods available from the natural environment[102]. It does not seem logical to advise populations away from carcass meat, dairy produce, eggs, nuts and seeds, in the name of saturated fat, when the modern processed foods, biscuits, cakes, pizza, desserts and ready meals, are more sensibly related to modern illness[73].

Close

An exchange between Dr Robert Olson of St Louis University and Senator George McGovern, chair of the Dietary Committee, was recorded in July 1977[103]. Olson said "I pleaded in my report and will plead again orally here for more research on the problem before we make announcements to the American public." McGovern replied "Senators don't have the luxury that the research scientist does of waiting until every last shred of evidence is in."

The evidence is now in. Indeed the evidence was available at the time. The original problem was defined in middle aged men. Middle aged men were the primary focus of RCTs and epidemiological evidence at the time: secondary men for the intervention trials and largely healthy men for the cohort studies. Despite only one study finding associations[3]; and many others advising caution[29, 31, 36] and despite a total lack of generalisability, guidelines were introduced for whole populations and have prevailed since.

An additional consequence of the guidelines is that, while it has been assumed that total and saturated dietary fat and dietary and serum cholesterol have been primary causes of CHD, factors of genuine concern have not been investigated as fully as they warrant.

The future will undoubtedly consist of the tailoring of diets and lifestyle to individual genomic makeup[104]. This will require the understanding of the genomic structure of circulating lipid profiles and replicable data on gene and diet interaction. Caution will be required in translating contemporary research on genes, diet and lifestyle into public health advice.

It is important that we learn from the study limitations and lack of evidence upon which current guidelines are based and not make the same mistake with future guidelines or suggestions.

Dr Zoë Harcombe, Ph.D

@zoeharcombe
zoeharcombe.com

Why Do You Overeat? When all you want is to be slim, Accent Press 2004 & Columbus Publishing Ltd 2013
The Obesity Epidemic. What caused it? How can we stop it? Columbus Publishing Ltd 2010
Stop Counting Calories & Start Losing Weight, Columbus Publishing Ltd 2011
The Harcombe Diet Recipe Book, Columbus Publishing Ltd 2011
The Harcombe Diet for men, Columbus Publishing Ltd 2011
The Harcombe Diet 3-step plan, Hodder Paperbacks 2013
The Harcombe Diet Lunchbox recipes, Columbus Publishing Ltd 2015
The Real Food Cookbook, Columbus Publishing Ltd 2016

Table 7.1 Summary of meta-analyses of RCTs and prospective cohort studies.

	Studies examined	Studies	People	Measure	Fat	Risk ratio	Conclusion
[63]	Prospective cohort studies & RCTs	28	280,000	CHD mortality	Total fat	0.94 [0.74, 1.18]	No sig difference
				CHD events	Total fat	0.93 [0.84, 1.03]	No sig difference
[62]	Prospective cohort studies	21	347,747	CHD fatal & non	Sat fat (Extreme quintiles)	1.07 [0.96, 1.19]	No sig difference
				CVD fatal & non	Sat fat (Extreme quintiles)	1.00 [0.89, 1.11]	No sig difference
[60]	RCTs	8	13,614	CHD events	Replacing SFA with PUFA	**0.81 [0.70-0.95]**	**Sig difference**
[59]	RCTs	21	71,790	Total mortality	All RCTs	0.98 [0.93, 1.04]	No sig difference
					Modified fat	1.02 [0.88, 1.18]	No sig difference
					Reduced fat	0.97 [0.90, 1.04]	No sig difference
					Reduced & modified fat	0.97 [0.76, 1.23]	No sig difference
				CVD mortality	All RCTs	0.94 [0.85, 1.04]	No sig difference
					Modified fat	0.92 [0.73, 1.15]	No sig difference
					Reduced fat	0.96 [0.82, 1.13]	No sig difference
					Reduced & modified fat	0.98 [0.76, 1.27]	No sig difference
				CVD events	All RCTs	**0.86 [0.77, 0.96]**	**Sig difference**
					Modified fat	0.82 [0.66, 1.02]	No sig difference
					Reduced fat	0.97 [0.87, 1.08]	No sig difference
					Reduced & modified fat	0.77 [0.57, 1.03]	No sig difference
[64]	Prospective cohort studies & RCTs	32	530,525	Coronary disease (All top vs. bottom third)	Sat fat	1.02 [0.97, 1.07]	No sig difference
					Monounsaturated fat	0.99 [0.89, 1.09]	No sig difference
					Polyunsaturated fat	0.93 [0.84, 1.02]	No sig difference
					Trans fat	**1.16 [1.06, 1.27]**	**Sig difference**

	Studies examined	Studies	People	Measure	Fat	Risk ratio	Conclusion
[58]	RCTs	12	7,150	All cause mortality	Modified fat intake	0.92 [0.68, 1.25]	No sig difference
				CVD mortality	Modified fat intake	0.96 [0.65, 1.42]	No sig difference
				CVD events	Modified fat intake	0.85 [0.63, 1.15]	No sig difference
				MIs	Modified fat intake	0.76 [0.54, 1.09]	No sig difference
				All cause mortality	Reduced fat intake	0.79 [0.42, 1.48]	No sig difference
				CVD mortality	Reduced fat intake	0.93 [0.66, 1.31]	No sig difference
				CVD events	Reduced fat intake	0.93 [0.65, 1.34]	No sig difference
				MIs	Reduced fat intake	1.18 [0.88, 1.59]	No sig difference
[23]	RCTs to 1977/1983	6	2,467	All cause mortality	Reduced or modified fat	0.99 [0.87, 1.15]	No sig difference
				CHD mortality	Reduced or modified fat	0.99 [0.78, 1.25]	No sig difference
[61]	RCTs	12	55,858	Total mortality	Reduced saturated fat	0.97 [0.90, 1.05]	No sig difference
				CVD mortality	Reduced saturated fat	0.95 [0.80, 1.12]	No sig difference
				CVD events	Reduced saturated fat	**0.83 [0.72, 0.96]**	**Sig difference**
				MIs	Reduced saturated fat	0.90 [0.80, 1.01]	No sig difference
				Non-fatal MIs	Reduced saturated fat	0.95 [0.80, 1.13]	No sig difference
				Stroke	Reduced saturated fat	1.00 [0.89, 1.12]	No sig difference
				CHD mortality	Reduced saturated fat	0.98 [0.84, 1.15]	No sig difference
				CHD events	Reduced saturated fat	0.87 [0.74, 1.03]	No sig difference

Table notes:

All studies examined data available at the time of the meta-analysis apart from Harcombe et al, which examined data available to the dietary committees.

Table 7.2 Study objectives and inclusion criteria.

	Objectives	Inclusion criteria
Skeaff & Miller (2009) [63]	To summarise the evidence from cohort studies and RCTs of the relation between dietary fat and risk of CHD.	Endpoints available for CHD deaths, events & total CHD. Dietary interventions: 1) change in poly/sat ratio 2) reduction in total fat 3) increase in fish intake 4) increase in n-3. No minimum length specified. Shortest study was 2 yrs follow-up. Adults.
Siri-Tarino (2010) [62]	Summarise the evidence for the association of sat fat with risk of CHD, stroke & CVD in prospective cohort studies.	1) sat fat intake available 2) endpoints for CVD deaths/events 3) association of sat fat with CVD evaluated 4) prospective cohort study 5) healthy adults at baseline. No min length specified. Shortest study was 5 yrs follow-up. Adults.
Mozaffarian (2010) [60]	Assess the effect of PUFA for SFA swap on CHD endpoints.	Increased total or n-6 PUFA; minimum 1 yr; reported sufficient data to calculate risk estimates for 'hard' CHD data – deaths/MIs. Adults.
Hooper (2011) [59]	Assess the effect of reduced &/or modified dietary fat on mortality, CVD mortality/ events & other outcomes (MI, stroke, cancer) in RCTs min 6 mths duration.	1) RCT 2) reduced or modified fat or cholesterol intake 3) not multi factorial, 4) adults with or without CVD 5) Min duration 6 months 6) mortality or CV morbidity data available.

	Objectives	Inclusion criteria
Chowdhury (2014) [64]	To summarise evidence about associations between fatty acids and coronary disease.	Prospective cohorts & RCTs that reported on associations of dietary fat intake, circulating fatty acids or fatty acid intervention with risk of CHD (fatal or nonfatal). Min 1 yr duration. Adults. Coronary outcomes as endpoints recorded.
Schwingshackl & Hoffman (2014) [58]	To investigate the effects of reduced and/or modified fat diets and dietary fatty acids on all-cause mortality, CVD mortality and CVD events in participants with established CHD.	RCTs comparing a modified or reduced fat diet vs control; min 1 yr duration; data on all-cause mortality, CVD mortality, CVD events and MIs available; secondary subjects only.
Harcombe (2015) [23]	Review dietary fat RCTs, with all/CHD mortality, at time of setting dietary fat guidelines.	RCTs that examined the relationship between dietary fat, serum cholesterol & mortality; available in 1983; min 1 yr duration; data on all-cause mortality, CHD mortality & cholesterol available.
Hooper (2015) [61]	Assess the effect of reducing sat fat intake & replacing it with carb, PUFA, MUFA &/ or protein on mortality and cardiovascular morbidity, in RCTs min 2 yrs.	1) RCT 2) reduced or modified sat fat intake 3) not multi-factorial 4) adult humans with or without CVD 5) Minimum duration 24 months 6) mortality or cardiovascular morbidity data available.

Table notes:

All studies excluded multi-factorial studies. The most common duration considered was a minimum of one year. Hooper 2011 included studies with a minimum of 6 months duration; Hooper 2015 included studies with a minimum of 24 months duration.

Chapter Twelve

Why do people with diabetes die from heart disease?

by Dr Jeffry Gerber, Ivor Cummins BE (Chem) CEng MIEI

Most diabetics die of heart disease, and they do so at a much earlier age than the average person. Diabetes is acknowledged as a powerful accelerator of cardiovascular complications, outweighing any other causal driver. Therefore, a book devoted to diabetes and its complications must cover this crucial area of risk.

For many decades the world of cardiovascular disease has centred on a person's 'cholesterol' levels as a causal driver. Supposedly the important parameter was the *quantity* of cholesterol trafficked in the blood. This could be the simple total, the amounts carried in LDL, HDL, or the amounts carried in other combinations of particles (called the 'lipoproteins'). More recently, the focus has moved towards assessing the number and size of the cholesterol-containing lipoproteins themselves. While the latter is more useful in predicting risk, it still fixates on 'cholesterol as cause'. However, we know that diabetes is a disease of insulin, glucose and metabolic/hormonal dysregulation. We also know that diabetes is a massive driver of cardiovascular disease, outstripping all other causes. So why do we still focus so much on 'cholesterol' in diabetes? Wouldn't it make much more sense to focus on the measures relating to *why* diabetes might drive cardiovascular disease? Why for instance does diabetes cause the 'cholesterol' to become problematic?

The reason we still focus on 'cholesterol as cause' is simply a matter of history. Cholesterol has always been perceived as the dominant driver of heart disease risk. The decades-long mainstream infatuation with it has tended to block out all other discussions. The cholesterol concept has been passed down from the medical authorities ever since it was first observed to accumulate as fatty streaks in the blood vessel wall. Unfortunately, this infatuation with cholesterol prevents most from recognising that heart disease is a complex metabolic disease. Many more important factors drive its progression. Although all the precise mechanisms are not yet fully understood, it is clearly a multi-factorial problem. Damage to cholesterol particles is just one step on the road – sadly viewed as practically the whole journey. The hormonal dysregulation of diabetes speaks to profound causes way beyond cholesterol. Insulin and glucose metabolism are accepted as key hormonal drivers. Failing to recognise the complexity and focusing on simply cholesterol is a tragically myopic approach.

Extensive literature review and clinical experience reveal that when it comes to addressing cardiovascular risk, cholesterol is mostly a *distraction* from the really important issues. Medical professionals feel that they are tackling the problem – while they are in fact missing the key measures. They are led astray from thinking about the real root causes. They are diverted from focusing on the far more crucial measures of the disease.

We will discuss insulin, hormonal dysregulation and metabolic disease later in this chapter. We trust that you will be fascinated to see the tapestry of real root-cause revealed. But first, let's review how the cholesterol distraction became rooted in our scientific and medical community. How did measuring cholesterol become the standard, and how did an intermediary piece of the problem come to be treated as the root cause in and of itself?

Lipid testing goes mainstream

Develop a new method and then build an industry around it. Most are familiar with the industry and the routine for lipoprotein measurement. You go to your doctor for a check-up and express concern about heart disease. The first test ordered by the doctor will be a standard lipid profile. Based on those results the doctor will provide standard advice including lifestyle, diet and sometimes medication. The primary goal will of course be to lower the 'bad cholesterol'. Depending on the doctor's level of knowledge, this could be LDL-C, TC or both. The perennial advice will then come forth: eat less, exercise more, reduce calorie-dense dietary fat, limit your saturated fat, etc. Medications will be strongly pushed if you are deemed anything above 'low risk'. This cholesterol-simplistic approach certainly makes the doctor's job easy. So how did we arrive with the one-factor wonder that is this 'cholesterol'? Let's take a brief look at the historical journey which led us to this surreal mono-focus.

Cholesterol is a 'sterol' molecule created by the animal world for myriad critical functions (plant-world sterols are called 'phytosterols). Trillions of cells are required for a human being to exist. Every one of these would fall apart without cholesterol. It is arguably the most vital molecule for life itself – no cholesterol, no life. Having been revealed as an identifiable substance in the 18th century, it was named via its discovery in bile and gallstones. So how did this important cholesterol get associated with potential problems? Well, the blood vessel disease known as atherosclerosis was widely recognised in the 19th century, but the etiology and clinical significance had yet to be established. Essentially, it was a problem waiting for a cause. Early in the 20th century, Adolf Windaus showed that atherosclerotic plaque, from the aortas of human subjects, contained higher concentrations of cholesterol than normal aortas; in effect, he was seeing a 20-fold increase.[1] Shortly after, Russian pathologist Nikolai Anitschkow fed pure cholesterol to rabbits, producing marked hypercholesterolemia and severe atherosclerosis in the aortas of these animals.[2] This was the first experiment showing a relationship between dietary cholesterol and atherosclerosis. It was exciting. The fact that this experiment was conducted in herbivores, fed a totally inappropriate animal-food cholesterol diet... was perhaps not seen as a major issue. Neither was the fact that the atherosclerosis observed was fundamentally different to that found in humans.

Cholesterol was measurable in the blood over the following years, yet further elucidation was lacking. Then in 1928 Michel Macheboeuf isolated a stable, water-soluble lipoprotein, now known to us today as the HDL. This complex macromolecule was capable of transporting water-insoluble substances including cholesterol and triglyceride in a water-based blood system. The extraordinary ingenuity of Mother Nature was revealed once again.

Following World War II (WWII), progress gained pace in the emerging field of lipidology. In 1949, John Gofman was to become known as the 'Father of Clinical Lipidology', due to his discoveries using ultracentrifugation techniques.[3] Beyond HDL, he further identified a family of lipoproteins (the sub-fractions). These included VLDL (very low density lipoprotein), LDL (low density lipoprotein), IDL (intermediate density lipoprotein) and others that are familiar to us today. He was in turn followed by Fredrickson, Gordon, Olson and Vester who identified specific lipoprotein *patterns* associated with atherosclerosis. Now there was a real excitement about 'cholesterol' as the causal agent in the world's most prevalent disease. Advances in measurement continued, including the deployment of chromatography and homogeneous assays. Lipid metabolism thus began to surge forward as a hot new science. It was the newest kid on the block, and the only one that had clear associations with the 21st century scourge of cardiovascular disease. By the 1970s and 1980s, standard lipid testing had become widely available to clinicians and patients. Everyone was all over the exciting new tools.

Cholesterol is the villain

Post WWII, the economy was booming and the new science was flourishing. Another thing that was flourishing, however, was the rate of heart attacks. In September 1955, the headlines were buzzing with news that the 34th president of the United States, Dwight D. Eisenhower, had been struck down with the new plague. At the age of 64, he had suffered a massive heart attack while on a golfing excursion outside Denver, Colorado. The stock market tumbled that day and heart disease became the hot topic, yet little was known as to its causes. The time was right to investigate. No one connected Eisenhower's heavy smoking habit with his heart event (smoking was not yet recognised as a massive driver of heart disease). So what could it have been? A suspect would have to be found – and convicted promptly.

Cholesterol quickly came under the spotlight. It was at the scene (in the atheromas themselves) – and it was also 'associated' with the crimes. With the rapidly advancing measurement technology came an opportunity to build further evidence against this new celebrity suspect. Driven by a few key researchers, a hypothesis emerged that was based mainly on the 'associational' data. The proposal was that elevated cholesterol in the blood was linked to higher risk of heart disease, and thus anything that might elevate cholesterol was likely to be a part of the problem. Quickly under suspicion became a diet high in natural saturated fats, as these were known to raise cholesterol in many (but not all) people. So beautifully simple and elegant was the theory, it gained many supporters. What held it back however, was an apparent built-in absurdity. How could an ancient human food, to which we arguably owe our very evolution, be the cause of a disease whose rate was now increasing rapidly in the 21st century? In spite of the logic issue, researchers, scientists, heart associations, national governments and the food and agriculture industry began to jump on board with the idea. They would be helped enormously in their conversion by the tireless work of an extraordinary individual named Ancel Keys. This influential researcher would near single-handedly gloss over the clear logic problem. He would generate a narrative that supposedly explained it all. The approach to cardiovascular risk assessment (and indeed dietary guidelines) would become a dogma destined to survive for decades. It would be a further half-century before logic and science could finally wrestle back control.

Artery clogging saturated fat – really?

Heart disease awareness and the war against cholesterol has dominated the nutrition landscape for generations. Membership of the 'Cholesterol Club' grew rapidly since the 1960s, with many in the nutritional field pursuing the relationship between dietary fat, cholesterol and heart disease. The new low-fat "diet-heart hypothesis" proposed that consuming dietary saturated fat would raise the bad cholesterol (TC & LDL-C) in the blood and so increase one's risk. Therefore, saturated fat should be reduced. The replacement should be polyunsaturated fats and/or carbohydrates. This simplistic solution would produce an 'optimal' lipid profile.

Between 1956 and 1958, researcher Ancel Keys began building on his previous work in this arena. He launched an epidemiological prospective longitudinal multi-country study to test this hypothesis. Named the Seven Countries Study, it became established as the de-facto proof of the hypothesis.[4] At the time, some scientists (and in recent years all well-informed ones), considered that it was actually one of the most misleading and flawed studies in scientific history.

Keys collaborated with lipoprotein pioneer John Gofman and received initial funding from the U.S. Public Health Service, the U.S. National Heart, Lung and Blood Institute and the American Heart Association. Persistent as well as persuasive, Keys passionately made his case against saturated fat. True, there was opposition from those who correctly challenged his methods, findings and also previous work. Keys had influence and connections, however, and successfully beat back the opposition. While scientist Professor John Yudkin from Europe was correctly focusing on sugar as a primary cause of chronic disease, his case was too late in being built (it was also fiercely fought against by sugar and food companies). With some sugar industry assistance, the anti-saturated fat campaign achieved enough momentum to steamroll over Yudkin's efforts.

By 1961, Keys had also achieved a key position on the nutrition committee of the American Heart Association. In testament to his enormous influence, he had even made it to the cover of Time magazine in recognition for his work. The American Heart Association had seen its funding increase massively during the heart attack 'crisis', and was becoming the most dominant force in the whole arena. Now it broke with tradition and made the first-of-its-kind dietary guidance to the government, and ultimately all of society. It came out and told everyone primarily... to reduce saturated fat in the diet.

The final monograph of Keys' Seven Countries Study was published in 1980, addressing the 'diet-heart' hypothesis.[5] It appeared to firmly convict dietary fat. Another parallel force was also convicting dietary fat for another crime, that of causing obesity. This was similarly based on a simplistic but false theory. Fat was higher per gram in calories than carbohydrate – so it had to be more fattening, right? There was no understanding of fat's hormonal and satiety-inducing effects however, so the framing of fat was delivered nicely. Both threads then came together in the perfect storm. Dietary fat would 'block your arteries' and also 'pile on the pounds'. However incorrect it was, the concocted logic was almost elegant. It made the following historical steps seem inevitable in retrospect. In 1977 a report was issued from The United States Senate Select Committee on Nutrition and Human Needs (infamously known as the McGovern report).[6] Although the Senate Committee did invite scientists who disagreed with the bad science, their voices were effectively ignored.

Thus in 1980 the first Dietary Guidelines for Americans (DGA) were published and enshrined in policy. They recommended a diet low in saturated fat for heart health and weight loss. They also suggested that a personal lowering of calorie intake was a good strategy for both aims. The world's nations followed suit with hardly a question. Notable was the 1983 dietary guidelines document published in the UK.[7] The DGA has since remained in place with minor updates every 5 years. In 2015 the current advice still restricts saturated fat to <10% of calories. In the US they have finally dropped the recommendation to limit total fat (and cholesterol) intake. However, the 'healthy alternatives' still include polyunsaturated fats, complex carbohydrates and naturally occurring sugars. Added sugars (refined and processed sugars) are currently suggested to make up <10% of calories.[8] Unfortunately, there was one notable and enormous unintended consequence from the whole DGA effort.

With the crystal-clear imperative to limit dietary fats, an enormous opportunity opened up to food companies. They would be able to fill the gap with 'healthier' substances. Unsurprisingly, the food industry did not fill the hole with broccoli and organic potatoes. Where would the profit be with that? You see, the mouth feel of natural fats was a key part of food consumption pleasure. It is difficult to replace this fundamental taste with anything comparable – but sugar was super-cheap and it really does the trick. And so it was that we entered an era of sugar, refined carbohydrate and industrial oils to replace our vilified ancestral foodstuffs. We can now look around at our fellow humans in any shopping mall, and wonder at the huge changes that have befallen them. We can openly observe what the disastrous DGA strategy has delivered.

So where's the evidence?

Distilling it down to its simplest form, the 'Cholesterol Club' had convinced everyone to fear saturated fat specifically and dietary fat in general. However, with the benefit of hindsight we can look back in history and ask a simple question. What specific scientific evidence genuinely supported this advice? Whatever claims were made about 'associations', 'hypotheses' and 'theories', one needs to prove them all *by running actual experiments*. You switch off (or lower) the supposed 'problem factor', and verify that the issue improves in real humans. So let's look at the human experiments that were executed. Did these experiments verify *any* of the theories?

Human feeding trials have been and always will be problematic and challenging, especially when it comes to looking at long-term outcomes such as cardiovascular disease. Imagine the difficulties: accurate food diaries, feeding compliance, controlling for every variable that might otherwise have an effect on health (confounding variables). You also need to monitor closely for outcomes over years or decades. These are called 'Randomised Control Trials' (RCT's), and they are real experiments that you can really prove things with. You would think that, with the health of the world's population at stake, they would overcome the challenges of such trials before implementing global dietary changes. However, they did not. In the end, they accepted Ancel Keys' population studies and similar 'associational' confections. These 'studies' were not RCT's – in essence they just tracked what people ate across different countries and what happened to them. They couldn't prove anything – especially when they were designed and executed in such a way that the eventual outcome could be hugely influenced. They indeed gave the answer that was desired, and the authorities ran with it. Statistically noisy and weakly associative data would be the only way to describe what they ran with.

Thus a clear relationship between total fat, saturated fat, cholesterol and heart disease had not been established. You would need RCT's for that. Interestingly, there *were* proper RCT's carried out in the period. Zoë Harcombe, Ph.D *et al* published a peer reviewed paper showing that all proper RCT experiments around the time of the Seven Countries Study *did not support the hypothesis*.[9] Harcombe concluded that there did not exist substantial evidence to support the recommendation to restrict dietary fat (total or saturated fat) in either the US or UK dietary guidelines before 1977 and 1983 respectively. They were running blind with what the President of the National Academy of Sciences, Phillip Handler, described as "a vast nutritional experiment conducted by federal government on the American people" (June 1980). Harcombe *et al* have also looked at the totality of RCT's carried out to date (many have been completed since the 1980s).[10] Shockingly, these also show that evidence does not exist to support present-day dietary guidelines, and that current guidelines

214

are in need of urgent revision. It turns out that the Emperor has been naked for 40 years, but nobody would call it.

So these are the dietary guidelines, which have been handed down to us on the low-fat plate, designed to supposedly reduce cardiovascular risk. The scientific evidence is certainly lacking, but the formula remains a misleadingly simple one: to reduce saturated fat in favor of polyunsaturated fats, complex carbohydrates and naturally occurring sugars. We will get back to our discussion regarding diet, but let us now make a visit to the area of risk assessment.

Diabetes and 'The Framingham Distraction'

It is well established in the medical literature, and with a growing body of scientific evidence today, that there is a strong link between diabetes and heart disease. However, this relationship is often overlooked when it comes to clinical medicine. The relatively rare, insulin-knowledgeable physicians (GPs) see this every day. Patients who are diabetic often are unaware that they have heart disease, while many heart patients don't know that they have diabetes. Even worse, their doctors are often clueless. This situation seems totally absurd, after decades of research and billions of dollars spent. One could well ask why this massive disconnect could be allowed to exist?

One answer to the previous question is what we call the "Framingham Distraction".[11] Framingham is a town in Massachusetts where a large population study was set in motion, with the unwritten goal of supporting the cholesterol hypothesis. Back in 1948, under the direction of Joseph Mountin from the US Public Health Service, Gilcin Meadors and colleagues began collecting population data. They were looking at epidemiologic factors associated with cardiovascular disease, the usual diet and exercise stuff. Importantly, they also tracked many blood test parameters including the darling data of cholesterol. In 1949, the study was transferred to the newly created National Heart Institute (later named the NHLBI) and, shortly after, Dr Thomas Dawber became the first director of the iconic Framingham Heart Study as we know it today. The Framingham Heart Study became a joint project of the National Heart, Lung and Blood Institute and Boston University.

Initially recruited were 5,209 people from the town who were followed over the decades, to see who experienced cardiovascular events and who did not. The recorded variables, which seemed to link to heart events, attracted a new terminology; they became increasingly referred to as "risk factors". Today, everyone is familiar with these risk factors. Some of the favourites are listed below:

- 'Bad Cholesterol' (LDL)

- Smoking

- Hypertension

- Diabetes

- Male sex

The Framingham Heart Study continues to this day and now covers six generations. Since the original work, various guidelines, tools and risk calculators have been spawned. All are designed around a central and singular theme: to lower the 'bad cholesterol'. Here lies the problem – it was decided in advance that cholesterol was the centre of the heart disease universe. With this dogma prevailing, everything else was forced to revolve around it.

We previously discussed the routine in the doctor's office, whereby the doctor asks a few questions related to risk factors and then checks the almighty lipid profile. This dated approach utterly fails to address atherosclerosis as the metabolic disease that it is. Fortunately, a more scientific approach has emerged in the past decade. It has been adopted by an increasingly large group of well-informed practitioners. It *does* recognise atherosclerosis as a complex metabolic disease, indeed one whose mechanisms overlap hugely with many others that are rampant in modern society. These others include diabetes / pre-diabetes / metabolic syndrome, but also extend to Alzheimer's, arthritis and many cancers. To address all of these maladies, one must focus on their common and most salient root causes. It goes without saying that 'cholesterol' is not one of them. As we advance, we realise that the primary root causes include inflammation, oxidative stress, advanced glycation, hormonal dysregulation, hyperinsulinemia and insulin resistance. We will discuss these further in the next section.

Framingham hardly addresses metabolic disease and the true root causes. A few questions are asked, blood lipids are measured and risk is then calculated based on epidemiological data. Epidemiology is great when looking at population risk, but using this type of data does not serve well when determining *individual* risk. Additionally, the risk calculators are heavily weighted towards a focus on 'bad cholesterol'. Although diabetes risk is represented, diabetes is not being properly measured in our current system. Bizarrely, insulin is not being measured at all. As a result, the contributions of metabolic disease including diabetes, pre-diabetes, hyperinsulinemia and insulin resistance are grossly underrepresented.

When it comes to determining individual risk, Framingham essentially takes a statistical guess. There is no fairer way of putting it. Overemphasising 'bad cholesterol', it weakly addresses the metabolic component of cardiovascular disease. Welcome to what we call the 'Muddy Waters' of Framingham. Through the murky soup of surrogate associative variables, they try to peer at each individual's metabolic health. This is a great disservice to each individual. They deserve better. Through measuring proper indicators of metabolic health, we replace the guessing game with solid scientific assessment. The individual deserves nothing less.

The cholesterol conundrum

The 'Cholesterol Club' has built an empire on the suspicion that elevated concentration of 'bad cholesterol' is associated with risk. It is almost as if they believe that cholesterol, the most vital substance for life to exist – is innately toxic. A simplistic mechanism that they use to support this hypothesis describes a 'concentration gradient' driver of vascular disease. If there are high numbers of cholesterol-filled lipoproteins in the blood, they will tend to burrow their way into your artery wall. Because of their specific size, they travel through the endothelial lining into the blood vessel wall. Here they automatically induce atherosclerosis. Carefully omitted from the simplistic theory is the idea that only damaged or 'oxidised' lipoproteins are problematic. We suspect the reason for the omission is also simple in nature – as it would beg the question *"what damages the lipoproteins though – surely **that** would be the root cause we seek?"* The latter question would of course lead us straight to the mechanisms of metabolic disease. Crucially, it would move us *away* from the simplistic 'bad cholesterol' theories. This we believe is the Cholesterol Club's greatest fear, as 50 years of dogma would begin to crumble. Thus we see little progress in the guidelines, in spite of the rapidly advancing science.

Why has the medical world advanced so slowly in this arena, in spite of the science? Is maintaining the status quo politically or financially driven? Or is it because people's reputations and egos are on the line, after generations hard-selling the misleading dogmas? The main hurdle with any new scientific discovery has always been dealing with obsolete approaches; as the late physicist Max Planck once said, "Science advances one funeral at a time". The challenge is particularly difficult in this area of science. It is generally accepted that the medical profession is an extremely conservative one, with scientific advances requiring 20 years or more to become established in practice. This particular example is even more fraught with difficulty – because there are enormous revenues and profit pools which are quasi-dependent on guarding the current dogmas. Luckily, the internet age is making it difficult to maintain the status quo. New generations of doctors are becoming research-savvy, and realising the profound mistakes of the past. They are no longer depending on being spoon-fed simplistic theories from their industry-funded organisations. They are networking across the world, and seeing past the Framingham distraction.

When we look closely at the physiology, atherosclerotic plaque is the result of a complex inflammatory process involving macrophages, foam cells and damaged/oxidised lipoproteins. True, the latter are derived from LDL cholesterol – but that is only an *interacting* player in the destructive milieu. We must see beyond the interacting agents and look to the root causes of the overall process. It is a progressive process whereby an initial insult to the blood vessel wall causes weakness, which attracts the body's healing components, just like any external cut or abrasion. Atheromatous plaque (atherosclerosis) simply represents the body's attempt to repair the damage, which by its nature recruits LDL cholesterol in the sequence. The biochemistry may be very complex, but it is bizarrely simplistic to implicate LDL cholesterol as causative by virtue of its presence. Hugely more important is to understand what factors are causing this initial damage. Equally important is to understand what factors lead to bad repairs and progressive instability of the plaques. Understanding metabolic disease provides the answers – whereas 'bad cholesterol' leads us down the garden path.

Atherosclerosis as a metabolic disease

As we said earlier, the causes of heart disease are quite complex, and a detailed discussion is not within the scope of this book. (Readers are recommended to read the "What causes heart disease?" series of blogs on Dr Malcolm Kendrick's site for a comprehensive exploration of factors that matter). Diabetes, however, is a primary driver of heart disease (arguably *the* primary driver). We will now reveal some realities around this epidemic affliction, and its super-accelerant role in heart disease progression.

We begin the story in 1988, long after the Framingham Heart Study and the Seven Countries Study had begun. This was the year that Stanford endocrinologist Dr Jerry Reaven delivered the Banting lecture, explaining to the world that heart disease was indeed due to metabolic dysfunction.[12] Reaven defined the root causes and pathophysiology. He demonstrated the central role of insulin resistance in Type 2 diabetes and cardiovascular disease. He also provided a practical approach to improve patient outcomes. He coined the term 'Syndrome X' to capture the broad dysfunction that was at the root of the diabetes and heart disease epidemic. He didn't fully realise at the time that the lion's share of modern inflammatory diseases were also connected to his syndrome.

Reaven's Syndrome X is today commonly referred to as the Metabolic Syndrome. The more correct term is Insulin Resistance Syndrome (for that is what it really is). Having the Metabolic Syndrome not only increases one's risk of developing cardiovascular disease but also appears to be linked to general chronic disease risk. Five major components are identified, which define insulin resistance as a pro-thrombotic and pro-inflammatory metabolic state:

- Hyperglycemia;

- Hyperinsulinemia;

- Atherogenic Dyslipidemia;

- Hypertension;

- Abdominal obesity.

Certainly there are genetic factors to consider, but these have not changed in the population during the past hundred years, during which our chronic disease rates have exploded. Based on the pathophysiology, the syndrome develops in response to energy overload from the diet. Insulin is a key hormone produced by the pancreatic beta cells, which not only regulates blood glucose but more importantly regulates and partitions energy between utilisation and storage. Insulin resistance develops after years of overconsumption. A vicious cycle develops as the body struggles to manage excess energy in a perpetual anabolic state. Excess energy can be stored as general body fat (subcutaneous) and/or as visceral fat (in and around the organs). The former is a relatively 'safe' way of dealing with excess energy, while the latter exacerbates metabolic disease. It is important to note that there are many non-obese people with metabolic dysfunction; although they appear ok, they have built stores of dangerous visceral fat in their organs – hidden and dangerous. While the insulin resistance grows, the end organ insulin receptors become increasingly resistant to the insulin signal. This in turn encourages hyperinsulinemia and drives the vicious cycle forwards.

Involved are many organ systems – primarily the liver, but also the pancreas, the adipose tissue, the gut and the central nervous system. Many other hormones become dysregulated in turn, and circulating inflammatory cytokines are produced from ever-increasing fat stores.

While Reaven focused on insulin resistance, it was pathologist Dr Joseph Kraft who decoded hyperinsulinemia and its implications.[13] During his career, Kraft performed five-hour insulin assays on a variety of patients – *over 16,000 people in total*. This extraordinary data, along with his extensive research on diabetes and heart disease, was profoundly revelatory. It revealed to him how diabetes and heart disease were inextricably linked together. Kraft thus identified the hyperinsulinemic state as a primary driver of metabolic disease; this in his opinion included the lion's share of cardiovascular disease in humans. Catherine Crofts, Ph.D has recently published new data based on Dr Kraft's work. She came to the same conclusions as Dr Kraft. She additionally detailed the mechanisms for hyperinsulinemia and metabolic disease.[14] In short, both hyperglycemia and insulin resistance are *late* findings to identify diabetic/metabolic dysfunction. Thus the people identified with diabetes have actually been diabetic for a long time – way before their eventual diagnosis. Thus their arteries have been assaulted continuously for many years (hyperinsulinemia's destructive processes care not about diagnosis status). Kraft stated that *"the vast majority of diabetics have no idea that they are diabetic – that is, until they have their first heart attack."* So we now understand that early screening is critical and should be the primary focus (a recent report showed that more than 50% of adult Americans have diabetic physiology). Unfortunately most healthcare professionals don't properly screen for hyperinsulinemia, hyperglycemia and insulin resistance. They wait for sky-high blood sugars to flag diabetes and metabolic disease. They are hopelessly distracted by the tired old 'bad cholesterol' cliché.

Atherogenic dyslipidemia

Atherogenic dyslipidemia is another important aspect of the metabolic syndrome, and serves as a simple proxy to insulin-centric determinations of metabolic health. Simply defined, it emphasises the importance of addressing the quality of lipoproteins, rather than just looking at cholesterol quantity (or concentration). Dr Reaven noted that certain lipoprotein patterns were closely associated with insulin resistance including low HDL cholesterol and high triglyceride. Today we can also measure the LDL particle size, (large favourable particles vs. small particles) providing yet another indicator that addresses cholesterol quality. By the way, LDL cholesterol concentration is not even considered relevant in determining if Metabolic Syndrome is present. It is not even worthy of measurement in the diagnosis. That in itself should tell you quite a lot.

The Framingham Heart study also recognised the importance of HDL, it being a marker inversely associated with mortality. Although this finding was published in 1988, it has been under-emphasised (probably as no drugs have been found to safely address low HDL). Thus the risk calculators still to this day emphasise addressing 'Bad Cholesterol', while HDL, the 'Good Cholesterol' remains a secondary goal. Additionally, while the Framingham data demonstrated a small association between LDL and mortality in younger adults, this relationship fell apart in older individuals. In fact, higher LDL was found to be associated with longevity in these older groups. This finding was not widely reported – as it challenged the entire 'Bad Cholesterol' theory.

Although most heart associations now recognise the metabolic syndrome, it is curious and disappointing that specific treatment related to the metabolic syndrome is not included in the current 2013 AHA guidelines. They seem to have an aversion to anything that relates to root cause, and prefer the soup of associational surrogates that overemphasises cholesterol as a primary target.

Metabolic mayhem

There are many contributors to heart disease progression, but the insulin resistance syndrome best describes the state that accelerates vascular degeneration. It is essentially a state of metabolic mayhem. Many organs and biological pathways are involved, as the body struggles to maintain homeostasis. All the while, a system-wide fire is burning through ones vascular network. What develops downstream is inflammation, oxidative stress and advanced glycation, which is ultimately damaging to multiple organ systems – especially the blood vessels. Within the blood vessels, atherosclerosis flares, and exposes the network to the risk of sudden ruptures. This is the genesis of most heart attacks.

It is important to recognise that atherosclerosis, atheroma or plaque, represents initially a protective mechanism. They seek to repair blood vessel wall damage. In a system experiencing metabolic mayhem, cholesterol and lipoprotein attempt an element of damage control. Tragically, lipoprotein-containing cholesterol also succumbs to the inflammatory forces. Becoming damaged itself, it furthers the disease process in ways. It becomes like the remaining jet fuel in a crashed airline. Where previously it was vital to keep the plane safely aloft, it now sadly contributes to destroying the surviving passengers.

So let us return to the question as suggested by the 'Cholesterol Club' – is cholesterol innately toxic? "No" says Uffe Ravnskov, Ph.D, who uses the analogy of cholesterol molecules as firemen at the scene of a conflagration: "It's as if they saw a house burning and determined that the bigger the fire, the more firemen are present, and then concluded that firemen cause burning houses." Also in agreement is Dr Malcolm Kendrick, a Scottish GP who has been researching this area for decades: "Essentially cholesterol is there to help repair damage. It's a bit like blaming firemen for causing fires, because they are there when fires break out." French biologist and author Sylvain Duval uses an analogy that is particularly useful. He suggests that LDL is like the ambulance going to the scene of an accident, while HDL is like an ambulance leaving the scene. We fixate on the ambulances while bypassing the root cause of accidents. Observations and associations can often be deceiving, and this is possibly the biggest case in scientific history where this has occurred. It is crucial to recognise and identify the true root causes, and not to be distracted by the interacting and confounded factors. Thankfully, the scientific and medical community are slowly waking up and perceiving the reality.

Atherosclerosis is a progressive process, and it is an unstable disease, which produces plaque most vulnerable to rupture. Quite revealing are the various *types* of plaque – including metabolically active soft, heterogeneous and the more stable calcific or hard plaque. Plaque can appear quite complex. For example some lesions have calcific caps and soft necrotic cores. The majority of acute cardiovascular events are due to the rupture of these vulnerable plaques, spewing out inflammatory substances into the blood vessel and causing sudden thrombosis. This is the acute coronary syndrome, a life-threatening condition that requires immediate intervention. If you are lucky enough to make it to the emergency room, thrombolytic therapy, angioplasty and or artery bypass might get you out of the immediate crisis.

Under these life-threatening circumstances everything else seems trivial, and the 'emergency plumbing work' is the order of the day. Yet proper screening for early subclinical disease would have been far more effective rather than waiting for the big event. Using tools, such as the heart calcium scan, to flag those exposed would greatly improve our accuracy in focusing on the right people. *Properly* addressing metabolic disease and the root causes would prevent millions from suffering and/or losing their lives. Whichever way you look at it, correctly addressing metabolic mayhem is the key.

It's the insulin stupid

As mentioned earlier, a recent study estimates that currently over half of the adult US population are pre-diabetic or diabetic (based on standard glucose testing).[15] Astounding as that number may seem, if we screened for hyperinsulinemia we would reveal an even larger problem. Many more would be flagged at risk and missed, if not tested in this way. Screening is important; yet sadly most healthcare professionals when thinking about cardiovascular disease do not measure glucose correctly. Also, they do not check insulin – nor is metabolic disease properly addressed.

Despite improved acute cardiac care services and smoking cessation, the occurrence of heart disease is still on the rise. It mirrors the rising incidence of diabetes and obesity. Although the linkage between diabetes and heart disease is well established, there is still a hurdle to overcome. We need to demonstrate that tracking metabolic disease better predicts risk, compared to simply looking at 'bad cholesterol' metrics. There are existing studies, including cardiovascular imaging and those that more properly measure glucose and insulin. When these are compared to studies looking at 'bad cholesterol', they show that glucose and insulin better predict cardiovascular risk.[16] Future research will most certainly support these mechanisms, but until that time properly addressing metabolic disease, hyperglycemia, hyperinsulinemia and the metabolic syndrome remains critical.

Atherosclerosis is a metabolic disease, which appears to be a consequence of hormonal dysregulation, hyperglycemia and hyperinsulinemia. Treatment by definition should therefore focus on metabolic disease improvement. Current medical doctrine and dogma have prevented us from doing this effectively.

The current approach favours a quick fix, be it medication and/ or procedures. The current approach is made very easy due to its leverage of the 'cholesterol is toxic' paradigm. When it comes to addressing metabolic disease properly, such simplistic approaches will not make the grade. Yes, you can still offer pills for reducing the effects of 'bad cholesterol', and even meds to mitigate the blood sugar problems. These approaches however, are still essentially band-aids on a rather nasty chest wound. To properly address the issue, we would need to explain the dietary root causes of the inflammatory milieu, to which people have exposed themselves. We would have to inform patients that the insulin resistance syndrome which afflicts them... has exclusively nutritional causes. We would have to convince them that there are genuine nutritional solutions, which are practical and feasible for them to implement. Of course, thanks to decades of low-fat anti-science, the public have little confidence in nutritional advice. They have seen the media coverage of the past few years – can we blame them for now being skeptical?

- Butter was bad, margarine was good – but now Time magazine and many articles say the opposite is true?

- Saturated Fat would clog your arteries – so, for heart health, we had to replace it with carbohydrates from the base of the food pyramid – but now the American Heart Association say that replacing saturated fat with carbohydrate *will give you more heart disease*?

- And so on, and so on – you've seen the daily headlines over the past few years.

This makes our job all the more difficult. The universally-supported low-fat and diet-heart myths have 'spoiled the pitch' for us all. How can we wrestle back the confidence of the average person in the nutritional solutions to their disease? Especially when many of the 'experts' still cling to the obsolete dogmas? This will be the primary challenge of the next decade. There is no question that insulin resistance syndrome is anything other than a nutritional syndrome, and that it is best addressed with diet (and also lifestyle). The diet should focus on driving down insulin, inflammation and metabolic disease (while simultaneously collapsing your cardiovascular risk). The low carbohydrate, high nutritional-density diet best addresses all of these aspects.

Low carbohydrate diets are unconventional and contradict the diet-heart hypothesis. That is the primary challenge facing their wide deployment. Although Dr Reaven and Dr Kraft knew of them, they chose not to challenge the medical orthodoxy. They felt that doing so would be pointless, given the sheer strength of the dogmas. They thus instead focused on their diagnostic methods, and proving what seemed now to be mechanistically obvious. A golden opportunity had been lost, but we cannot blame them for holding back on the full truth; they would have been ostracised and undermined for doing so. Thankfully today (with more scientific evidence available), low carbohydrate diets are gaining momentum. There is hope that this quasi-obvious tool in combating diabetes will become the standard of care.

A well-formulated, nutrient-dense low carbohydrate diet addresses the full spectrum: diabetes; heart disease; and metabolic disease. High insulin load foods, containing simple carbohydrates from sugars, grains and starches, promote inflammation and must be limited. Protein intake remains moderate, but varies based on age and activity. Natural fats (including mono and saturated) appear to be metabolically neutral, are healthy to consume and help with satiety. Refined and processed foods including the highly atherogenic industrial vegetables oils such as Canola, Soy and Corn must be restricted. Nutrient density of foods and overall food quality are also very important. The types of foods that we eat have a direct effect on our appetite control system through hormonal regulation; thus the correct diet can greatly help with weight loss efforts too. Eating the right foods will enable us to eat less in general, and recent science is connecting this to long-term anti-aging benefits. There is much more to consider including movement and activity, smoking cessation, proper sleep, stress reduction, etc. Low carbohydrate diets however, are a very appropriate starting point.

Clinical assessment addresses metabolic disease and cardiovascular risk. An early and high level of suspicion is what's most important. Healthcare professionals need to address metabolic disease and screen for overweight, obesity, pre-diabetes, diabetes and hyperinsulinemia. Inflammatory markers can be measured, as well as lipids; however, it is cholesterol *quality*, not just the *quantity* that is important. Cardiovascular imaging using tools like the heart calcium scan would be a powerful addition, as it has the ability to actually *see* sub-clinical disease.

There has been more than half a century of scientific progress since the 1960s, and yet the 'Cholesterol Club' still dictates their dogmatic approach to the problem of cardiovascular disease. It now appears totally outdated, and is a distraction from the real issues. Advancing science recognises that atherosclerosis is a complex metabolic disease, which has causes way beyond (and far more important than) cholesterol. In medicine, we had better wake up and understand these root causes, and how to appropriately take action to resolve them. If this is achieved, we, and all medical professionals, could see clearly beyond the muddy waters of Framingham. Our medical professionals would see that diabetes and cardiovascular disease are two sides of a dysfunctional coin. Most importantly they would finally internalise... *that diabetes is a vascular disease.*

Dr Jeffry Gerber*, Ivor Cummins BE (Chem) CEng MIEI**

* *@jeffrygerbermd*
denversdietdoctor.com

** *@fatemperor*
thefatemperor.com

Chapter Thirteen

Why are low carbohydrate high fat diets best for all persons with Type 2 Diabetes Mellitus and for almost all athletes?

Professor Timothy David Noakes OMS, MBChB, MD, DSc, Ph.D (hc), FACSM, (hc) FFSEM (UK), (hc) FFSEM (Ire)

Summary

According to current medical and dietetics practice, athletes and persons with Type 2 Diabetes Mellitus (T2DM) are both encouraged to eat low fat high carbohydrate (LFHC) diets to ensure their health and optimum athletic performance. But the question is not often asked: What if the LFHC diet promotes the development of T2DM even in active individuals? And what if the LFHC diet worsens the prognosis of those with T2DM?

In this chapter I provide the experimental evidence which shows that humans, most especially those with insulin resistance and T2DM, have no essential requirement for carbohydrate. This is because the human liver is more than capable of producing all the glucose required to maintain blood glucose concentrations even in those eating diets with very low carbohydrate content. Next I show that the single most important determinant of the blood glucose concentration is the amount of glucose delivered to the portal vein following the intestinal digestion and absorption of ingested carbohydrate. Logically then, the simplest method to regulate the blood glucose concentration in those with either normal or impaired (T2DM) whole body glucose metabolism, is simply to restrict the amount of dietary carbohydrate ingested each day to ~25 g.

I further argue that these data strongly suggest that humans are not biologically adapted to the ingestion of high (>200 g/day) carbohydrate diets on a regular (chronic) basis. This is because *Homo sapiens* evolved from omnivorous primates whose survival was dependent on the ability of their gut microbes anaerobically to produce volatile fatty acids (VFAs) from ingested carbohydrate (cellulose). As a result liver glucose production from VFAs is the sole source of circulating blood glucose in herbivorous mammals as would have been the case for those primates from which humans evolved. And not from ingested glucose appearing in the portal vein as is now the case in those humans eating high carbohydrate diets.

I next discuss the popular belief that all athletes need to ingest high carbohydrate diets to optimise their athletic performance, regardless of the duration, intensity or frequency of their activities. At present the evidence appears to be the following: For higher intensity exercise of short duration, for example single day running races of 400 m to 42 km (marathon), the best performing athletes still prefer to eat more carbohydrates, sometimes in very high daily amounts (>500-600 g/day). When the exercise is prolonged with intermittent bouts of high intensity and extends over many days or weeks, as occurs for example in the Tour de France cycling race, the best performers are steadily moving away from exclusively high carbohydrate diets. But carbohydrates continue to be ingested both before and during the longer race stages, most especially when sustained effort of very high intensity is to be expected, for example in the mountain stages.

When the exercise is intense but intermittent as in team sports like football or rugby, for example, other benefits of the LCHF eating plan – for example lesser hunger, better weight control, more rapid recovery from exercise, perhaps fewer injuries and illnesses – may become equally important determinants of match-day performance. As a result over the past two to three years, some elite football and rugby teams have begun a discernible movement away from exclusively high carbohydrate diets and towards diets based on "real foods".

But when the activity is more prolonged, for example greater than three hours, the lower exercise intensity allows stored body fat to provide the majority of the energy. Thus ~73% of the energy used during an 8-hour Ironman Triathlon will come from fat oxidation in a fat-adapted athlete, with minimal requirement for ingested carbohydrate. In this and similar events it is clear that performance is determined by the ability to use fat, not carbohydrate as the "King" fuel.

In contrast a carbohydrate-dependent athlete would theoretically need to ingest ~1 kg of carbohydrate to maximise performance during that same race. This raises an important question that has been overlooked: Does the ingestion of so much carbohydrate daily over years or decades promote long-term health? Based on our current understanding one might suggest that whilst such a high carbohydrate intake may indeed be "safe" for those who are insulin-sensitive, for the insulin-resistant majority, such a high daily carbohydrate load must over a period of decades, worsen insulin resistance, likely leading ultimately to T2DM.

The over-riding conclusion from this chapter is that for both recreational athletes and for those with T2DM, the optimum diet for physical activity and for long term health is the same. It is a diet that minimises daily blood glucose and insulin excursions by limiting the delivery of glucose to the portal vein. To achieve this the diet must be restricted in its carbohydrate content and consequently higher in dietary fat.

By producing the state of fat-adaptation in which essentially all the energy for daily living comes from stored body fat, this diet also ensures that the energy needs of physically-active recreational athletes can also be provided almost exclusively from body fat stores.

Introduction.

For 33 years I personally ate and promoted a high carbohydrate diet for both health and for athletic performance. So in the 4th Edition of my book *Lore of Running*[1] published in 2002, I wrote that: "... all athletes ... must be advised to eat high-carbohydrate diets both in training and especially before competition ... this interpretation forms the central pillar ... (of) the profession of sports nutrition ... as high carbohydrate diets are now considered ideal for both health and sport." I no longer believe that this statement is correct. In fact I now think this advice is totally wrong and probably harmful to a majority of those who might choose to follow it.

My moment of personal truth came in December 2010 when overweight and struggling to run with anything even approaching enthusiasm, I chanced upon the book, *The New Atkins for the New You*[2], written by Drs Westman, Phinney and Volek. Within two hours of opening the book for the first time, I realised the extent of the error that I had made for more than three decades. By following these three

231

mavericks' "controversial" advice to remove most of the carbohydrate from my diet so that I now eat 25 g carbohydrate/day or less, and by returning to the foods on which my Lancashire (Liverpool) parents had raised me first in Zimbabwe and then in South Africa, my body weight dropped to what it had last been as an athletic medical student in the early 1970s.

In time I would also discover that despite running a total of 70 marathon/ultramarathon races and eating the specific heart-healthy, prudent, low fat diet "in moderation" that the experts had assured would make me the epitome of cardiovascular health, I still managed to develop Type 2 diabetes mellitus (T2DM). This I ascribe to ingesting too much sugar and too many carbohydrates for too many years in my genetically-predisposed state, shown by a very strong family history of T2DM – my father dying from the condition and various other aunts and uncles on both sides of my family, also developing the condition. Data from a research trial I participated in in 1978 when I was in my late twenties show that I was then already profoundly insulin resistant with pathologically elevated fasting blood insulin concentrations when "carbohydrate loading" for marathon racing[3].

Following this low carbohydrate high (healthy) fat (LCHF) diet proposed by Dr Westman and his colleagues for 6 years, has unfortunately not "cured" my T2DM. But together with exercise and daily doses of metformin and berberine, my glucose control has not deteriorated during that time so that my most recent set of blood tests were all in the normal range. Not measured by these results would be the beneficial effects of 6 years of low daily blood insulin concentrations produced by the LCHF diet. For it seems highly likely that in those with T2DM, it is chronically elevated blood insulin concentrations either self-injected or as the result of eating high carbohydrate diets that produces that widespread organ damage that is the quintessential feature of this potentially devastating disease[4].

This personal experience has focused my attention on the physiopathology of T2DM and how best it should be managed. Understanding this pathophysiology explains, in my opinion, why the current management protocols do not improve long-term outcomes in T2DM[5]; instead they likely aggravate the condition.

Here I wish to present the important biological principles that, in my opinion, determine the macronutrient composition of the diet that

232

persons with T2DM should be eating and how or why that diet might be the same or different for those who are habitually active, either as elite or recreational athletes.

Point 1: Humans (and most especially those with insulin resistance and T2DM) have no essential requirement for carbohydrate.

A key argument used to explain why persons with T2DM must ingest carbohydrates in large amounts on a daily basis is, we are told, because, like all humans, those with T2DM need to fuel their brains since "the brain is dependent on glucose for its energy metabolism".

According to this logic, persons with T2DM who fail to eat sufficient carbohydrate will suffer from impaired brain function and presumably long-term brain damage. This statement is falsified by (i) the existence of human populations like the Inuit[6] and the Masai who remain healthy despite ingesting little carbohydrate; (ii) the ability of humans to survive protracted periods of starvation; an unavoidable state that would have happened countless times in the three million years it took for modern humans to evolve from our ancestral hominins so that (iii) the very existence of the human race disproves this implausible statement.

The biological evidence that falsifies this statement is the following:

First, the blood glucose concentration is regulated by the human liver which has the capacity to produce all the glucose required to maintain that concentration, regardless of how much dietary carbohydrate or glucose is ingested. It does this by generating (new) glucose from other dietary precursors, in particular protein and fat in the process known as liver (hepatic) gluconeogenesis.

Second, whilst the brains of individuals eating high carbohydrate diets utilise glucose at about 5 g/hr, this is an extravagance. Instead the brain has an essential glucose requirement of only about 1 g/hr[7] that must come from glucose and cannot be provided by alternate fuels. Since the maximum glucose generating capacity of the healthy liver is about 25 gm/hr and is ~6 g/hr at rest even in those who ingest no carbohydrate (see later – Figure 3)[8], there will never be an occasion when the healthy liver cannot maintain an adequate glucose delivery to the bloodstream and hence to the brain. The sole exception is when normal rates of liver glucose production are prevented by excessively high circulating insulin concentrations in those injecting insulin for the (inappropriate) management of T2DM or Type 1 diabetes (appropriate).

Third, the human brain has the capacity rapidly to adapt its metabolism to utilise ketone bodies[7] and lactate as alternate fuels should dietary carbohydrate intake fall even to zero in those who are either fasting, or starving or eating no carbohydrate diets.

Fourth, persons with T2DM have elevated blood glucose concentrations – the diagnostic feature of the disease. This is because of uncontrolled excessive liver glucose production. Thus there is never any possibility that those persons with T2DM (who do not inject insulin and who are therefore at no risk of developing insulin-induced hypoglycemia – see later) will ever be at risk of providing their brains with too little glucose.

I have yet to understand why those who give dietary advice that persons with T2DM need to ingest carbohydrate to "protect their brains" fail to understand that the characteristic feature of T2DM pathophysiology is an overproduction of glucose by the liver under all circumstances. So if they were logically consistent, those who currently prescribe high carbohydrate diets for those with T2DM should have concluded long ago, that T2DM patients do **not ever** need to ingest carbohydrates to ensure their brains are receiving an adequate glucose delivery. The pathology of their disease always ensures that there will be more than enough blood glucose to fuel their brains (presuming they do not over-dose on insulin).

Fifth, persons with T2DM do not die because their livers are unable to provide sufficient glucose to maintain the health of their brains. They more usually die from disseminated obstructive arterial disease leading to heart or kidney failure or peripheral gangrene. My interpretation is that it is the prescription of high carbohydrate diets for persons with T2DM and the resulting chronic hyperinsulinemia that is the direct cause of this arterial disease[4].

To study how the liver adapts to a LCHF diet we recently reported a study[8] of 14 athletes, 7 of whom had adapted to a LCHF diet by eating less than 50 g carbohydrate/day for more than 8 months. The 7 matched control athletes ate a conventional high carbohydrate diet providing more than 50% of daily calories as carbohydrate for an average daily carbohydrate intake of more than 350 g. Our key question was to determine if and how persons eating so little carbohydrate (by modern standards) are able to regulate their blood glucose concentrations both at rest and during prolonged exercise. To answer this we specifically studied rates of liver glucose production from either stored liver glycogen (glycogenolysis – the breakdown of stored glycogen) or from gluconeogenesis (the production of new glucose from precursors including lactate and glycerol) at rest and during exercise. The key findings are shown in Figures 1-5.

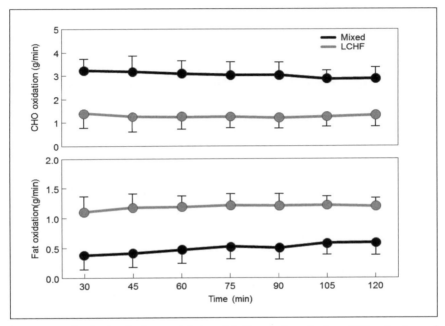

FIGURE 1 Carbohydrate and fat oxidation rates during 120 minutes of exercise in subjects eating either mixed or LCHF diets. Redrawn from Reference 8.

Figure 1 (top panel) shows that during exercise subjects eating the high carbohydrate diet oxidised about 3 g/min of carbohydrate during 120 minutes of exercise (total ~360 g) whereas rates of carbohydrate use in the LCHF group were <1.4 g/min (total ~160 g). Thus athletes on the LCHF diet "spared" about 200 g carbohydrate during the 120 minutes exercise bout, a saving of ~55%. As shown in the bottom panel of Figure 1 this sparing was achieved by the much greater contribution of fat oxidation to overall metabolism in the LCHF group. Thus the top line in that panel shows that the average rate of fat oxidation during exercise in the LCHF group was ~1.2 g/min whereas athletes eating the high carbohydrate diet achieved a peak fat oxidation rate of only ~0.5 g/min at the end of exercise. Notably high rates of fat oxidation were present from the start of exercise in the LCHF athletes whereas rates rose progressively in athletes eating the high carbohydrate diet.

Thus athletes eating a high fat diet are "primed" to burn fat at high rates even from the moment they begin exercise.

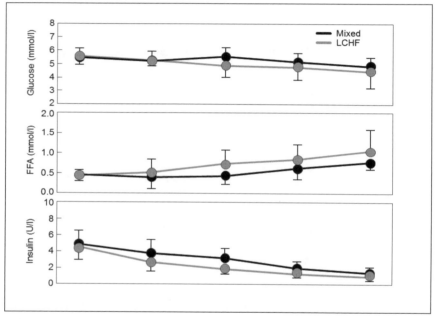

FIGURE 2 Changes in blood glucose, free fatty acid (FFA) and insulin concentrations during 120 minutes of exercise in subjects eating either mixed or LCHF diets. Redrawn from Reference 8.

Figure 2 (top panel) shows that blood glucose concentrations were similar in both groups and remained in the normal range throughout exercise. As expected, circulating free fatty acid (FFA) concentrations rose during exercise (middle panel) but were also not different between groups. Similarly blood insulin concentrations (bottom panel) were low; they fell during exercise and were not different between groups. Thus the 140% greater rates of fat oxidation in the LCHF athletes cannot be explained by higher circulating FFA concentrations resulting from lower circulating insulin concentrations producing a lesser inhibition of fat mobilisation. Instead the increased capacity of the fat-adapted athletes to use fat as a fuel must have been due to skeletal muscle adaptations favouring fatty acid oxidation[9].

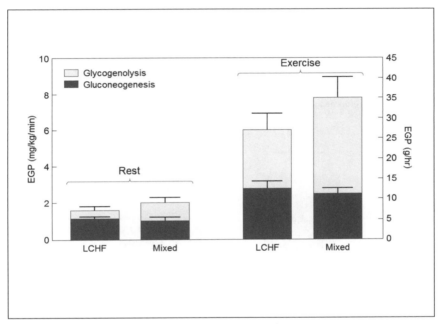

FIGURE 3 Endogenous glucose production (EGP) rates from glycogenolysis and gluconeogenesis at rest (left columns) and during exercise (right columns) in subjects eating either mixed or LCHF diets. Redrawn from Reference 8.

Figure 3 shows the rates of endogenous glucose production (EGP) from glycogenolysis (breakdown of previously stored glucose) and gluconeogenesis (production of new glucose from protein and fat precursors) in the subjects at rest (left panel) and during exercise (right panel). At rest, rates of EGP were about 25% higher in athletes eating the high carbohydrate diet (right column) due to higher rates of glycogenolysis. Exercise caused a marked three to four times increase in EGP in both groups of athletes with higher rates again in those eating the high carbohydrate diet. Higher EGP rates were achieved in both groups by marked accelerations in rates of both glycogenolysis and gluconeogenesis. Importantly the higher EGP rates in athletes eating the high carbohydrate diet were achieved by larger increases in glycogenolysis; the contribution from liver gluconeogenesis was marginally but not significantly higher in subjects eating the LCHF diet both at rest and during exercise.

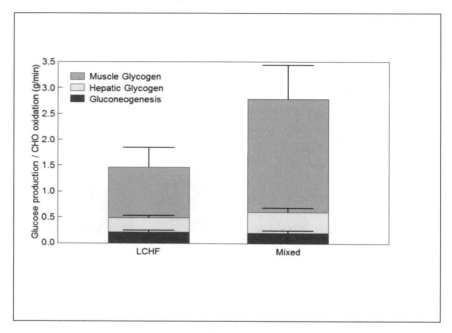

FIGURE 4 Glucose production/oxidation rates from muscle and liver glycogen stores and from liver gluconeogenesis during exercise in subjects eating either mixed or LCHF diets. Redrawn from Reference 8.

Figure 4 shows the origin of the glucose used during the 120 minutes of exercise by athletes eating the LCHF (left column) or the high carbohydrate diets (right column). The much higher rates of glucose use by athletes eating the high carbohydrate diet are explained mainly by higher rates of muscle glycogen and to a lesser extent liver glycogen use. These would be the result of much higher muscle and liver glycogen stores at the start of exercise in those eating high carbohydrate diets.

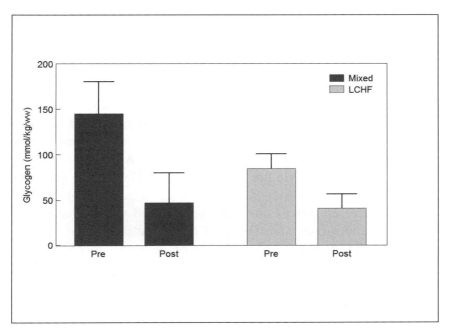

FIGURE 5 Muscle glycogen contents before and after 120 minutes of exercise in subjects eating either mixed (left columns) or LCHF (right columns) diets. Redrawn from Reference 8.

Indeed Figure 5 shows that at rest, muscle glycogen concentrations were approximately twice as high in athletes eating the high (left panel) compared to the low carbohydrate diet (right panel). However at the end of exercise, muscle glycogen concentrations were the same showing the much reduced contribution of muscle glycogen to energy metabolism in fat-adapted athletes.

So this study confirms the following:

- Humans adapt to the LCHF diet by dramatically reducing their dependence on carbohydrate for energy production. They achieve this by a very large increase in their capacity for fat oxidation.

- Humans eating the LCHF diet regulate their blood glucose concentrations as effectively as do those eating high carbohydrate diets. They achieve this by (i) dramatically increasing rates of fat

239

oxidation with a large overall reduction in whole body glucose use; and (ii) by maintaining normal or slightly elevated rates of liver gluconeogenesis.

- At rest, humans eating the LCHF diet continue to generate glucose endogenously at rates of up to ~6 g/hr and can increase this to up to ~27 g/hr during exercise (Figure 3). At rest any endogenously produced glucose that is not used immediately as a fuel will be stored in muscle and liver. As a result athletes eating LCHF diets do not have "zero" muscle or liver glycogen stores. Instead muscle glycogen stores in athletes eating the LCHF diet are about one-half those found in athletes eating high carbohydrate diets (Figure 5). The realisation that athletes eating the LCHF diet do have substantial muscle glycogen stores becomes important when we consider the potential effects of the LCHF diet on physical performance especially during exercise of higher intensities.

- Humans have no essential requirement for carbohydrate or at least beyond 50 g/day as shown in this study. This is compatible with the conclusion of the Institute of Medicine[10] that: "The lower limit of dietary carbohydrate compatible with life apparently is zero, provided adequate amounts of protein and fats are consumed" (p. 275).

Thus the essential paradox that we face in the management of T2DM is simply stated:

The single macronutrient that persons with T2DM have great difficulty metabolising and for which neither they nor any other humans appear to have any essential requirement is the macronutrient that current T2DM dietary guidelines propose must provide up to 50% of daily energy intake or about 300 g/day.

The next point explains what the ingestion of that 300 g/day does to blood glucose control in those with and without T2DM.

Point 2: The single most important determinant of the blood glucose concentration is the amount of glucose delivered to the portal vein following intestinal digestion and absorption of ingested carbohydrate.

The blood glucose concentration is tightly regulated by a range of exquisite, complex homeostatic processes that in health ensure a stable concentration of about 5 mmol/L. In persons with T2DM ingesting little carbohydrate (less than 25 g/day) the same applies – the blood glucose concentration is also homeostatically regulated but at a concentration higher than 5 mmol/L. So the homeostatic set point for the blood glucose concentration is probably elevated to between 6.0 and 7.0 mmol/L in those T2DM patients who have relatively the best good glucose control (because they are eating an LCHF diet and using appropriate medications, but not insulin).

The point is that homeostatic control of blood glucose still exists in those with T2DM. The reason most practitioners and patients do not realise this is because the very obvious evidence for this homeostatic control is obscured by frequent erratic oscillations in blood glucose concentrations in those whose daily carbohydrate intake is much more than ~25 g/day; that is one-sixth of the carbohydrate intake currently prescribed for persons with T2DM.

What is perhaps most clearly ignored by proponents of high carbohydrate diets for all is just how little carbohydrate exists freely in the human bloodstream in both the healthy and in those with T2DM. In a healthy individual a normal blood glucose concentration of 5.0 mmol/L represents 0.9 g glucose/L of blood for a total of just 4.50 g in the total blood volume of 5 L.

In contrast a person with T2DM who maintains an average blood glucose concentration of 6.5 mmol/l will have, on average, a total of 5.85 g of glucose in her blood stream.

Thus T2DM occurs when the 5 L blood volume of the average human contains 1.35 g more glucose than it should.

Yet official dietary advice encourages persons with T2DM to eat at least 300 g of carbohydrate/day. What is the probability that eating so much carbohydrate every day for decades plays at least some small part in first causing and then sustaining that 1.35 g glucose excess in the bloodstream of those with T2DM?

And what if the tiny amount of free carbohydrate in the bloodstream indicates that humans were never really meant to eat much carbohydrate?

My logic for arguing this untested hypothesis is the following:

First the manner in which the human body handles ingested and digested fats and carbohydrates is fundamentally different. Whereas carbohydrate enters the bloodstream directly following digestion and absorption in the small intestine, initiating a rapid hormonal response, fat does not initially enter the bloodstream. Nor does it trigger the same hormonal response.

Instead the intestinal cells repackage digested and absorbed dietary fats into chylomicrons which are then transported by the lymphatic drainage system – the lacteals – to the venous bloodstream (via the thoracic duct) entering a short distance from the superior vena cava that travels directly to the right side of the heart. In this way ingested fat travels through the right side of the heart to the lungs before it travels via the arterial blood circulation to all organs in the body, including the liver. The key point is that unlike ingested carbohydrate which, when absorbed, goes directly to the liver in the form of glucose, ingested fat is initially delivered to all the organs in the body, not just to the liver.

Interestingly microbial activity in the voluminous intestines of herbivorous mammals, like cattle and antelope, ferment the ingested carbohydrate (cellulose) anaerobically into volatile fatty acids (VFAs), predominantly acetic, proprionic and butyric acid[11, 12]. As a result whilst superficially these mammals appear to be eating high carbohydrate diets, in fact they are eating diets high in fat, most of which is saturated. Most of the ingested protein is also metabolised to VFAs by microbial activity. As a result "from the standpoint of the host animal, VFAs are the important product of fermentation. These small lipids are used for many purposes but the paramount importance of VFAs to herbivores is that they are absorbed and serve as the animal's major fuel for energy production..."[11] "providing greater than 70% of the ruminant's energy supply"[12].

Bowen[12] continues: "Let's put some of this academic information presented here into perspective. The little goat pictured here weighed about 200 lb when this picture was taken and produced 1570 kg of milk in a 305-day lactation. Her milk was roughly 4% lactose,

242

3.5% protein and 3.6% fat. This means that, for the sole purpose of producing milk, this goat had to synthesise about 250 grams of lactose and 180 grams of protein and 185 grams of fat every day".

"*Essentially all the glucose in that lactose was synthesised in the liver* and most of that synthesis was from propionic acid generated by fermentation. Likewise, much of the fat was synthesised from ruminant acetate. When you consider the synthesis of lactose and milk fat are only two of many, many processes that are supported by VFAs, the process of fermentation in herbivores gains new meaning".

But what is crucial for our understanding is that **the liver of ruminants generates the glucose they require from VFAs. As a result ruminants are not ever exposed to high blood glucose concentrations following the ingestion of their high carbohydrate (cellulose) diets (as now occurs in modern humans ingesting readily digested carbohydrates, whether "low" or "high" GI (glucose index) every few hours).**

The end result is that all mammals subsist on high fat diets. The sole exception is humans after we were advised to adopt high carbohydrate diets by the 1977 US Dietary Guidelines!

The point, of course, is that humans evolved from omnivorous but predominately vegetarian primates that also ate high carbohydrate diets, the digestion products of which (following microbial fermentation in their voluminous large intestines) would also have been predominantly VFAs, not glucose.

But sometime in the past 3 million years of our evolution, our hominin ancestors developed the intestinal characteristics of carnivores, losing the spacious fermenting large intestines present in modern primates and whose function is to convert ingested carbohydrate into VFAs. As a result our hominin ancestors had to develop alternate mechanisms to deal with the more rapidly digestible carbohydrates found especially in roots, bulbs, fruits and honey that constituted a (small) part of their predominantly carnivorous diet.

My suggestion is that evolutionary pressures during those three million years were never sufficiently stringent to force our common *Homo sapiens* ancestor that arose in Africa about 200,000 years ago, fully to have made that transition. So my conclusion is that the hominins leading to *Homo sapiens* did not ever eat sufficient carbohydrate on a daily year-round basis to require the development of safe biological pathways to handle high glucose loads entering the portal vein every few hours, as has now become the feeding pattern of the majority of living *Homo sapiens*, especially since publication of the 1977 US Dietary Guidelines.

That the livers of modern primates are not properly designed to maintain blood glucose homeostasis when fed high carbohydrate diets is clearly established by the fundamentally important study of Fabbrini and colleagues[13]. They were able to measure what is not possible in humans, specifically the effects on (endogenous) liver glucose production (EGP) of additional glucose entering the liver directly from the intestine.

For their experimental model, the authors surgically implanted a cannula in the portal vein (which carries absorbed nutrients from the intestine to the liver) in a group of omnivorous (occasionally carnivorous) primates (baboons). They then used radio-labelled tracers to measure the rates at which glucose was "appearing" (i.e. entering or fluxing into the blood in the portal vein flowing from the intestine towards the liver) and the rate at which glucose was "appearing" from the liver into the systemic circulation for distribution to all the organs of the body. They were also able to measure liver EGP rates from gluconeogenesis and glycogenolysis.

On two separate occasions the baboons were fed either a high (65%) carbohydrate low fat (HCLF) meal made from crushed brown rice krispies, glucose powder, butter and whey protein isolate or a low (20%) carbohydrate high fat (LCHF) meal prepared from butter, smooth peanut butter, honey crackers, whey protein, and dextrose.

Their findings are shown in Figure 6.

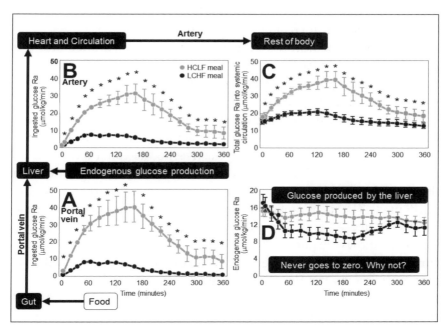

FIGURE 6

A. Ingested glucose Rate of Appearance (RA) in the portal vein in primates fed either a high carbohydrate (top line) or a low carbohydrate (bottom line) meal.

B. Ingested glucose Rate of Appearance (RA) in the systemic circulation in primates fed either a high carbohydrate (top line) or a low carbohydrate (bottom line) meal.

C. Total (ingested and endogenous) glucose Rate of Appearance (RA) in the systemic circulation in primates fed either a high carbohydrate (top line) or a low carbohydrate (bottom line) meal.

D. Endogenous glucose Rate of Appearance (RA) in the systemic circulation in primates fed either a high carbohydrate (top line) or a low carbohydrate (bottom line) meal.

All redrawn from Reference 13.

The bottom left panel (A – Portal vein) shows the rates of appearance of (ingested) glucose absorbed from the intestine into the portal vein following ingestion of either the HCLF (top curve) or the LCHF (bottom curve) meals. This ingested carbohydrate is also termed exogenous as it originates from outside the body; endogenous carbohydrate is that glucose that is generated within the body. The portal vein carries ingested carbohydrate from the intestine to the liver.

Note that the peak rate of ingested glucose appearance into the portal vein is at least four times higher from the HCLF than from the LCHF meal and peaks three hours after the HCLF meal but much sooner after ingestion of the LCHF meal.

Panel B shows the rate of ingested glucose appearance from the liver into the blood circulating to the rest of the body. Note that the rate of ingested glucose appearance from the liver to the general circulation is still much higher following the HCLF meal but once passing through the liver, the increase is only about three times higher than from the LCHF meal. This is because of extraction of about one-quarter of the ingested glucose for metabolism or storage (as glycogen) by the liver.

Panel C shows the rate of total (endogenous and ingested/exogenous) carbohydrate being released by the liver; once more the value is greater following the HCLF meal. Note however that the peak rate of total glucose appearance following the HCLF meal (~40 mmol/kg/min) is not different from the rate of ingested glucose appearance which is approximately the same value.

This is because the ingestion of the HCLF meal produces a large reduction in EGP (Panel D) between 60 and 120 minutes following meal ingestion. This effect will be driven by much higher rates of insulin production following the HCLF meal as insulin is the key inhibitor of EGP through its action in inhibiting glucagon production (as glucagon is a key driver of EGP). But the lesser release of insulin in response to the ingestion of substantially less carbohydrate in the LCHF meal will have a much smaller effect on EGP (bottom curve in Panel D).

Thus there are at least two key observations from this study.

First that the rate of exogenous glucose absorbed from the intestine is the key driver of meal-induced changes in the blood glucose and insulin concentrations (not shown). This is high when a HCLF meal is ingested and low when a LCHF meal is eaten (Panel A).

Second, in contrast, the relatively unchanged rates of total glucose appearance (Panel C) regulate the blood glucose concentrations and as a consequence, the blood insulin responses to the LCHF meal. This is so because when little carbohydrate is ingested from the LCHF meal, EGP is appropriately reduced (Panel D) (with minimal insulin secretion) so that total glucose appearance remains relatively unchanged.

My interpretation is that the primates studied in this research have, like humans, not ever evolved to ingest rapidly absorbed carbohydrates in amounts that produce high rates of ingested glucose appearance into the portal vein. Because if they (and we) had indeed developed those adaptations, the ingestion of carbohydrate in these amounts would produce an *immediate and complete suppression* of EGP. The effect of this evolutionary biological adaptation (that did not ever happen) would have been to ensure that blood glucose concentrations do not rise whenever carbohydrates are ingested. (There does not seem to be any benefit achieved by a meal-induced increase in the blood glucose and insulin concentrations, only potential harm as discussed subsequently).

Instead Panel D in Figure 6 shows that this adaptation has not developed. Instead EGP drops to rates that are only about 50% of resting values continuing at high rates (of about 2 mg/kg/min equivalent to about 9 g/hr in 70-80 kg humans – essentially the same as values we measured in resting humans eating high carbohydrate diets – Figure 3) even in the face of a torrent of glucose appearing in the portal vein. This failure of complete suppression of EGP results from a failure to inhibit glucagon production sufficiently (data not shown). But for what purpose is it necessary for the liver to continue producing glucose at 50% of resting (fasting) rates when so much glucose is already present in the portal vein?

For at that time the rate of (total) glucose appearance into the bloodstream (Panel C) is at least twice as high following ingestion of the HCLF than the LCHF meal. The end result will be that after ingestion of the HCLF meal all the tissues in the body will be exposed to an excess of circulating glucose. We now know that high circulating blood glucose concentrations produce damage, especially to proteins, in the process of glycation[14].

So none of this makes any biological sense. It is clearly a serious human biological flaw that will be exposed whenever humans choose to eat carbohydrates in amounts greater than those to which our hominin ancestors were accustomed.

The point is that if humans (and primates) had been designed differently, a high carbohydrate meal would have triggered a massive insulin response with complete suppression of glucagon secretion producing an immediate reduction in (unnecessary) EGP[15]. As a result the blood glucose concentration would not rise in response to carbohydrate ingestion. This is clearly possible when little carbohydrate is ingested as occurred in the LCHF section of this experimental primate study. But equally obviously, there must be a threshold carbohydrate intake above which this does not happen. Instead EGP continues in excess causing blood glucose concentrations to rise, leading to at least some of the toxic consequences we see in those with T2DM.

In summary, this study shows that when little carbohydrate is ingested as in the case of the LCHF meal in this experiment, the blood glucose concentration will remain essentially unchanged and will be determined by the background rate of EGP by the liver and its partial suppression by the insulin released in response to the small amounts of carbohydrate (and protein) in the meal. In contrast the blood glucose concentrations of those eating HCLF diets, whether or not they have T2DM, will be determined by the (average) rates of ingested glucose appearance in the portal vein – in other words by the amounts of carbohydrate they eat each day.

So we can logically conclude that in persons with T2DM eating LCHF meals, it is their inherent rates of EGP that will be the key determinant of their blood glucose concentrations. Or stated differently: If we wish to control blood glucose concentrations in those with T2DM we have to minimise their rates of **total** liver glucose production (from the combined effects of ingested glucose added to the background rates of EGP). This is most effectively achieved by insuring (i) that they eat very little carbohydrate (Panel C) and that (ii) their EGP is minimised by interventions aimed at increasing the effectiveness of the biochemical processes by which insulin inhibits glucagon production in the pancreas (and perhaps elsewhere).

Interestingly, this study's authors concluded that: "Our data demonstrate that in adult male baboons a LCHF meal elicited a less robust insulin secretory response compared with a HCLF meal and support the importance of further studies to assess the potential for therapeutic benefit of a low-carbohydrate diet on glycemic control and prevention of Type 2 diabetes".

Not that too many Diabetes Associations around the world have yet taken much notice of this conclusion.

But hope springs eternal!

Point 3: Surely carbohydrates are essential for exercise, even in those with T2DM?

The reason why I and others fell in love with carbohydrate as the key drivers of exercise performance was a group of studies[16] conducted in the 1960s which apparently showed that endurance exercise performance was determined by one factor, specifically the extent to which the muscle glycogen stores are filled at the start of exercise (Figure 7). The beauty of such simplistic, reductionist thinking is that it dramatically simplifies teaching and research in the field. Who needs to think when we already have such a simple solution? Especially if our research was being funded by an industry that rewarded us for believing in this simple paradigm (as did my industry funding at the time).

So for a (very long) period all we needed to do in our research programs was to measure muscle glycogen content and to tell athletes to eat as much carbohydrate as possible to maximise their performance. Fortunately we now know that humans are complex organisms; their exercise performances cannot be so simply explained[17].

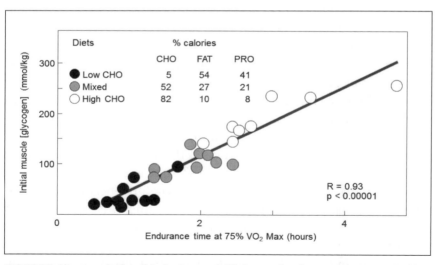

FIGURE 7 Linear relationship between initial muscle glycogen concentration and endurance time at 75% VO2 max in subjects eating either low, mixed or high carbohydrate diets. Redrawn from Reference 16.

Figure 7 purports to show that there is a linear relationship between muscle glycogen concentrations at the start of exercise and the duration for which exercise of moderate intensity can be sustained. This "evidence" was all that was required to launch a global industry providing cheap, highly refined carbohydrates (with long shelf-lives) to athletes for use before, during and after exercise. The associated marketing convinced and continues to convince most of the world's exercisers that when it comes to exercise, carbohydrates are "King" whereas fat is an inferior exercise fuel. For some of us with a genetic predisposition (perhaps relating to the mechanisms described in Point 2), this advice is probably the key driver causing us to develop T2DM as did I and as have some "real" athletes like Sir Steven Redgrave[18], indisputably one of the very greatest Olympic athletes of all time. Like me Sir Steven also has a family history (grandfather) of T2DM.

After so many years of this uncontrolled marketing hyping "King Carbs", it is perhaps unrealistic to expect many immediately to change their belief in the central importance of carbohydrates for exercise performance.

In retrospect the evidence from these studies was anything but conclusive. In the first place the studies were poorly controlled, in particular, they did not include any placebo interventions. Secondly the LCHF diets needed to produce the low muscle glycogen concentrations were followed for very short periods usually about three days. In 1984 Phinney and colleagues[19] showed that humans require a period of at least 3-6 weeks properly to adapt to the LCHF diet.

But in 2000 we published the first[20] and one of very few placebo-controlled studies of carbohydrate-loading. The study failed to show any benefits of carbohydrate-loading; in hindsight it is perhaps surprising that the paper ever made it through peer review since it provided evidence that was so contrary to the dogma of the day. I would personally require another 10 years before I began to question whether our annoyingly inconvenient finding was real and was not, as we had tried to explain away at the time, an artifact of some experimental design flaw.

Our "pro-King Carbs" bias was strongly influenced by another study we published in 2006[21]. This study became known as the final "nail in the coffin"[22] for those promoting LCHF diets for athletes.

For that study the same group of athletes completed two 100 km laboratory cycling time trials, one on their normal high carbohydrate diet and the other after eating an LCHF diet for 6 days. To re-stock their muscle glycogen stores athletes ate a high carbohydrate diet for the final 24 hours before both trials. Overall performance was *not* influenced by the dietary intervention, a point which has tended to be ignored. Figure 8 shows the "nail in the coffin" problem that we uncovered.

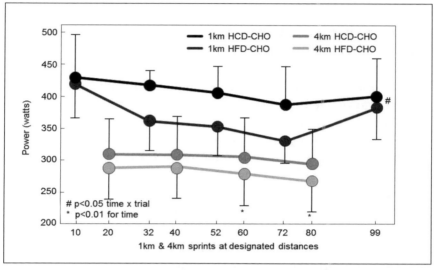

FIGURE 8 **Power outputs in cyclists during successive 1-km (upper 2 lines) and 4-km intervals as part of two 100-km time trial in subjects who ate either high carbohydrate diets for 6 (plus 1) days (HCD-CHO) (top lines in both series) or a high fat diet for 6 days followed by 1 day of a high carbohydrate diet (HFD-CHO) (bottom lines in both series).**

The upper lines in that figure show the power produced by athletes during 5 one-km sprints performed at specific intervals during the overall 100 km time trial; the lower set of lines records their power outputs during 4 four-km sprints also performed at specific distances during the time trial.

The lower pair of lines shows that there was no difference in power outputs between dietary groups during the 4-km sprints. However average power output during the 1-km sprints was significantly lower after the LCHF diet. Accordingly we concluded that the LCHF "dietary strategy increased fat oxidation, but compromised high intensity sprint performance, possibly by increased sympathetic activation or altered contractile function".

Again in hindsight, this conclusion is itself suspect. For the reason that the power outputs in the last of the five 1-km sprints were identical in both groups. This indicates that the lower power outputs in the second to fourth 1-km sprints in the LCHF group was not because those subjects were "metabolically crippled" and unable to produce the necessary metabolic energy. For that to be true, power production during the fifth 1-km sprint should also have been lower.

Rather this pattern shows a different pacing strategy following the LCHF diet. This in turn indicates a central brain effect[17] – in particular a more conservative pacing strategy – as might be expected in athletes who had never before performed such a time trial after eating an LCHF diet for 6 days.

More recently Burke et al[23] have indeed shown that elite athletes attempting to train vigorously for three weeks on an LCHF diet do not improve their performance in a subsequent ~40 minute time trial whereas athletes eating high carbohydrate diets during the same period improved their performances by about 5%. This finding is consistent with reports of many elite athletes that the LCHF diet impairs exercise performance during high intensity exercise of short duration; supportive of the finding reported in Figure 8.

We[24, 25] have recently reviewed the published evidence which suggests that eating an LCHF diet is more likely to be beneficial during more prolonged exercise lasting three or more hours, as well as for the long-term health most especially of those with insulin resistance.

For example a simulation of the metabolic requirements of running a 2 h 40 min 42 km marathon at the end of the 242 km Ironman Triathlon[1] (pp. 141-143) argues that carbohydrate-adapted Ironman triathletes with extremely low muscle glycogen concentrations at the start of the final 26.2 mile marathon run, would require a minimal fat oxidation rate of 1.15 g/min to complete the marathon in 2 h 40 min when the carbohydrate contribution to energy production (from the oxidation of blood glucose (~1.2 g/min) and lactate (~0.6 g/min)) could provide ~31.5 kj/min or less than about 43% of the total rate of energy expenditure (74 kj/min) required to maintain that running speed.

Although the highest rates of fat oxidation we measured in the fat-adapted athletes in our study[8] were in this range (~1.2 g/min) (Figure 1), the studies of Volek et al.[26] and Burke et al[23] measured peak rates of fat oxidation of 1.5 g/min or even higher.

252

An Ironman athlete able to oxidise fat at a rate of 1.5 g/min would be able to produce 56 kj/min from fat oxidation alone or 73% of the 74 kj/min needed to run a 2 h 40 min Ironman marathon. This leaves just 18 kj/min to be provided by the oxidation of glucose and lactate. We have measured rates of lactate disappearance from the bloodstream of between 0.7-1.4 g/min[27] which would provide between 12-25 kj/min if all the lactate "disappearing" were fully oxidised.

More recently Emhoff et al[28] measured slightly higher rates of lactate appearance (1.8 g/min) during exercise at the "lactate threshold". They also showed that 86% (1.5 g/min) of the lactate "disappearing" was directly oxidised, providing 26 kj/min.

Thus these data show that a fully fat-adapted but muscle-glycogen depleted athlete can theoretically fuel a 2 h 40 min marathon at the end of an Ironman triathlon from the oxidation of fat and lactate alone without even requiring additional glucose derived from liver gluconeogenesis.

Accordingly, provided the fully fat-adapted athlete was able to provide as little as 18 kj/min from lactate and glucose oxidation, he or she should be able to provide sufficient energy to run at that pace without requiring any external source of feeding.

In reality many fat-adapted athletes report that they benefit from ingesting some carbohydrate during exercise lasting more than three or so hours. This would be explained if their combined rates of lactate oxidation and of liver EGP were unable to cover the small carbohydrate requirement of those fat-adapted athletes.

But the real point is the following: Even if these athletes are ingesting carbohydrate, the vast majority of their energy (~73%) is coming from fat oxidation. Of course this is an inconvenient fact that the purveyors of the "King Carbs" dogma will not ever acknowledge.

For example how does one justify the statement that: "When the exercise is more prolonged (2 h or more), carbohydrate becomes a very important fuel, and to prevent a decrease in performance it is essential to ingest carbohydrate"[29]. The reality is the opposite – the longer the duration of the exercise, the greater is the contribution that fat makes to energy production after five or more hours of continuous exercise.

In summary, I would agree that at present the published evidence strongly suggests that at least for the very best athletes involved in short duration high intensity exercise, high carbohydrate diets seem to produce the best performances[30].

So for higher intensity exercise of short duration, for example single day running races of 400 m to 42 km (marathon), the best performing athletes still prefer to eat more carbohydrates, sometimes in very high daily amounts (>500-600 g/day). But when the exercise is prolonged with intermittent bouts of high intensity and extends over many days or weeks, as occurs for example in the Tour de France cycling race, the best performers are gradually moving away from exclusively high carbohydrate diets. Thus the two top performers in the 2016 Tour de France, Chris Froome[31] and Romain Bardet[32], both reported that they were eating fewer carbohydrates and more fat than has been the Tour de France tradition[33, 34]. But carbohydrates continue to be ingested both before and during the longer stages, most especially when sustained effort of very high intensity is to be expected, for example in the mountain stages.

When the exercise is intense but intermittent as in football or rugby, for example, other benefits of the LCHF eating plan – for example lesser hunger, better weight control, more rapid recovery from exercise, perhaps fewer injuries and illnesses – may become equally important determinants of match-day exercise performance. As a result a discernible movement away from exclusively high carbohydrate diets by some elite football and rugby teams has happened over the past two to three years[35, 36].

An interesting question is: How might intensive intermittent exercise be unchanged on a high fat diet whereas sustained exercise of a similar intensity seems to be impaired?

Hetlelid and colleagues[37] have recently shown that when performing 6x4 minute intervals at maximal effort (87-94% maximum oxygen consumption – VO_2 max), recreational and well-trained athletes achieved identical rates of perceived exertion, blood lactate concentrations and rates of carbohydrate oxidation. However the much faster running speeds and higher exercise intensities (94% VO_2 max) achieved by the well-trained athletes were associated with approximately threefold higher rates of fat oxidation. Furthermore in contrast to the conventional teaching that fat oxidation does not contribute to energy production during exercise at intensities >85% VO_2 max, fat oxidation provided nearly one-third of the total energy expenditure in these well-trained athletes when they ran at maximal effort repeatedly for four minute intervals. The authors concluded that: "The greater capacity to perform high-intensity intermittent work is mostly explained by the higher fat oxidation rates in well-trained runners".

Perhaps it is not entirely improbable that exceptional athletes involved in high-intensity intermittent sports like rugby and soccer might achieve that status in part because they also have a superior capacity to utilise fat as a fuel during this type of exercise.

But it is very difficult to argue that, once the activity lasts more than three or more hours so that muscle glycogen depletion inevitably develops, a high carbohydrate diet is definitely the best for all, regardless of their athletic abilities.

TABLE 1: **Energy metabolism during an 8-hr 242 km Ironman Triathlon compared in carbohydrate- and fat-adapted athletes.**

Variable	Carbohydrate-adapted athlete	Fat-adapted athlete
42 km marathon time (hr:min:sec)	2:40:00	2:40:00
Oxygen consumption (ml/kg/min)	53	53
Energy cost (kj/min)	74	74
Fat oxidation rate (g/min)	0.5	1.5
Energy from fat (kj/min)	19	56
Energy from carbohydrate (kj/min)	55	18
Energy from carbohydrate (g/min)	3.3	1.1
Total carbohydrate use during 8 h Ironman Triathlon (g)	1584	528

For example consider the case of a carbohydrate-adapted athlete trying to run a 2 h 40 min Ironman marathon when his peak rate of fat oxidation is only 0.5 g/min (Figure 1). To provide the additional 55 kj/min required to run at that pace would require a carbohydrate oxidation rate of 3.3 g/min (Table 1). If this applied for the entire duration of the race, the carbohydrate-adapted athlete would oxidise a total of 1584 g carbohydrate during an 8-hour Ironman triathlon whereas a fat-adapted athlete would oxidise less than 33% of this amount (528 g) (Table 1).

Since the total carbohydrate stores in an elite 70 kg Ironman triathlete are probably of the order of 500-600 g[1], this would require the carbohydrate-adapted athlete to ingest close to 1 kg of carbohydrate during the race. (Hepatic gluconeogenesis would contribute about 100 g of glucose during the 8 hours of the race (Figure 3).

Perhaps this is why the advocates of high carbohydrate diets suggest that Ironman triathletes must ingest carbohydrate at rates of up to 90 g/hr during these events (Total of 630 g for 7 hour combined Ironman cycle and run legs)[29]. The fact that many are able successfully to complete Ironman triathlons without ingesting anywhere near this amount of carbohydrate suggests that these athletes are perhaps far more fat-adapted than the promoters of the "King Carbs" dogma ever care to acknowledge.

But how healthy would it be to ingest 630 g of carbohydrate during 7 hours even if one was exercising vigorously?

Point 4: Is it really safe to eat a 50-60% carbohydrate diet even if one is highly active?

My personal experience and that of "real" (world-class) athletes like Sir Steven Redgrave suggests that perhaps eating all that carbohydrate may not be such a good idea in the long term.

Indeed the real problem with studies comparing low and high fat diets for athletes[22, 24, 25, 30] is that the outcome measure in all these studies is simply performance in a single laboratory or field exercise trial. As a result, in our review of the published evidence comparing the effects of athletic diets with different macronutrient contents, we specially lamented the absence of studies "addressing the effects of low-carbohydrate diets on the ease of weight control in athletes, on their capacity to train and their ability to recover, on their immune function and injury risk, or on their hand-eye coordination or capacity to concentrate in sports like golf and cricket, to name but a few obvious research questions. Clearly there is still much to be done"[24]. Especially missing are studies of the potentially detrimental effects of ingesting perhaps 500-1000 g of carbohydrate daily for decades by elite athletes.

Dr Philip Maffetone was one of the first scientists of whom I am aware who was promoting LCHF diets especially for ultra-endurance athletes already in the 1980s[38]. He was a major influence on the Ironman Triathlon careers of Mark Allen and Paula Newby-Fraser, both of whom dominated their sport for more than a decade whilst eating more dietary fat than was then considered appropriate. Allen won six Hawaiian (World Championship) Ironman Triathlons and Newby-Fraser eight. The third great six-time Hawaiian Ironman champion of that era, David Scott who, in contrast, then ate the more conventional HCLF diet, has since also converted to a higher fat diet and has written: "A high-fat diet is superior to a high-carb diet. One of the benefits is that it helps you recover faster"[39]. Scott now reports that he eats a 60% fat, 25% protein and 15% carbohydrate diet. During exercise he ingests an amino-acid solution and eats mixed nuts and coconut flakes[40].

I have always wondered if the very long and successful professional careers of Allen and Newby-Fraser might perhaps be best explained by their adoption of the higher fat diets during their athletic careers. Their long careers perhaps provide anecdotal evidence that requires proper scientific investigation.

Mark Allen was certainly in no doubt of the importance of this dietary advice on his own career for he subsequently wrote[41]: "During my 15-year career as a professional athlete, the attention I gave to diet was critical to my success. Initially what I ate was swayed by the athletic diet *du jour*. Most of the fad diets were based on bad science that had nothing to do with sustaining performance over time in the real world. Fortunately, I met Dr Phil Maffetone, who coached me to eat according to what the body actually needs and responds to in training and racing".

"The best part of his dietary guidelines is that they followed the balance of my body's natural cravings. There was nothing that went contrary to the voice of my body telling me what to eat. This was very different than my experience with other diets and eating regimens".

"The results speak for themselves. I was able to sustain a world-class level in a very demanding endurance sport for 15 years, winning 6 (Hawaiian) Ironman Triathlon titles along the way" (p. 7).

Mike Pigg, who won four US National Championships at the Olympic distance triathlon, also paid tribute to the benefits of this diet program: "The ideal (Dr) Phil (Maffetone) presents are off the beaten track and can be found in no other nutrition book on the market. Not only will you find this book helpful in improving athletic performance, it also offers solid ideas in improving health, losing weight and increasing energy"[42] (p. 9).

"Over the last century humans have gotten farther and farther from their evolutionary diet. We evolved as hunters and gatherers, but now most people eat like feedlot cattle. I noticed that in my own dietary evolution I began to reach for whole foods rather than processed ones, especially refined carbohydrates. I increased my protein intake by eating more meat and eggs. I seriously took stock of my carbohydrate intake, relying mainly on fruit, fresh or steamed vegetables and small amounts of whole grains. I also increased my consumption of healthy fats by adding more avocados, butter, nuts and seeds to my diet. My increased fat and protein intake has given me more energy".

Recently Maffetone and Laursen[43] have suggested how a diet high in refined carbohydrates may contribute to ill-health in vigorously training athletes. A subsequent case study[44] of a 38-year-old professional triathlete reported that her symptoms of decreased performance, severe gastrointestinal distress, excessive fatigue and hunger were eliminated when she converted from a 73% to a 12% carbohydrate diet and reduced her training load. This intervention also produced new personal best times.

I have also made the point[45] that the unexpected presence of coronary artery disease in some habitual marathon runners[46] might be linked, not to their choice of exercise, but perhaps to diets high in sugar, refined carbohydrates and, I would now add, perhaps vegetable oils.

These reports are interesting but they do not provide answers about the long-term health effects of combining very intensive training with eating high carbohydrate diets.

My impression is that the final answers will come from the athletes themselves[31, 32, 35, 36, 39-44].

Point 5: So what is the best dietary advice for the average athlete including those with T2DM?

Here I think the evidence is very simple – eat a diet of those real foods[47] that are optimum for long term health, which in my judgement is a real food diet that minimises daily fluctuations in blood glucose and insulin concentrations by limiting the delivery of glucose to the portal vein (Figure 6). This diet will be low in carbohydrate and consequently high in (healthy) fat with a moderate protein content.

This eating pattern produces a state of fat adaptation in which the person's body fat stores alone can fuel any type of recreational physical activity without the need for energy supplementation (except perhaps if the activity lasts more than two to three hours).

And what of the athlete with T2DM? Is not the T2DM athlete at risk for the development of hypoglycemia during exercise?

Recall that the key abnormality in T2DM is the persistent overproduction of glucose by the insulin-resistant (and glucagon-overstimulated) liver. This overproduction likely continues during exercise. Perhaps the key reason to promote exercise for persons with T2DM is to offset this excess production by increasing peripheral glucose use thereby temporarily depleting liver and muscle glycogen stores with exercise. This will allow increased post-exercise glucose storage in liver and muscle, temporarily improving blood glucose control.

I am unaware of any studies of blood glucose regulation during exercise in persons with T2DM eating an LCHF diet. My prediction, based on my personal experience and discussions with others with T2DM also eating LCHF diets, is that it is almost impossible for persons with T2DM to develop symptomatic hypoglycemia even when eating very low carbohydrate diets. The reason, in my opinion, is that exercise alone is unable to reduce glucose overproduction by the diabetic liver to the point at which it falls dangerously below peripheral glucose uptake, potentially causing hypoglycemia. Rather it is injected insulin and not a low carbohydrate diet that causes symptomatic hypoglycemia in T2DM. And my experience is that, provided they follow the LCHF eating plan, persons with T2DM can effectively control their blood glucose concentrations without the need to use insulin.

As a result the only persons with T2DM who need to be cautious when exercising are those who continue to eat high carbohydrate

259

diets and who as a result may need to inject insulin to keep their blood glucose concentrations within some measure of control.

In those injecting insulin either T1DM or T2DM the problem is that insulin absorption from the injection site appears to increase during exercise leading to hyperinsulinemia; whereas normally exercise causes blood insulin concentrations to fall.

As a result: "Even in the presence of high levels of all the counter-regulatory hormones, a high free insulin level is a powerful inhibitor of glycogenolysis, gluconeogenesis and lipolysis[48]. In the hyperinsulinaemic state, muscle glucose uptake is unimpaired but glucose mobilisation is low and the muscle deprived of glucose cannot simply shift to burning fat."

"Therefore, exercise should occur not necessarily when blood glucose levels are high, but when free insulin levels are low"[49] (p. 804).

The same author makes the additional important point that: "In the normal subject, the hormonal response to exercise is geared not to stimulate glucose uptake by the contracting muscle but to mobilise fuel for the contracting muscle[50, 51]" (p. 803), the latter by ensuring that blood insulin concentrations are as low as possible.

Which is perhaps just one more good reason to maintain low blood insulin concentrations whenever possible (by following a LCHF eating plan).

Professor Tim Noakes

@proftimnoakes
thenoakesfoundation.org
Lore of Running, Human Kinetics 2002
Waterlogged: The serious problem of over hydrating in endurance sport, Human Kinetics 2012
Challenging Beliefs: Memoirs of a career, Struik Publishers 2012
The Real Meal Revolution: The radical sustainable approach to healthy eating, Robinson 2015
Super Food for Superchildren: Delicious, low-sugar recipes for healthy, happy children, from toddlers to teens, Robinson 2016
The Banting Pocket Guide, Penguin 2017

Chapter Fourteen

The politics of nutrition

Nina Teicholz

This book has presented a robust body of scientific evidence to make the case that a low-carbohydrate diet should be considered at least one, if not the best, approach for treating Type 2 Diabetes.[1] Given the global failure to make any meaningful progress to date in combating this type of diabetes, one has to ask why this new and promising approach has not been more enthusiastically embraced by health officials. In fact, we see quite the opposite, with authorities in quite a few countries attempting to shut down those practicing or promoting a low-carbohydrate approach. These events cannot be described as routine disciplinary actions. They appear instead to be oppressive attempts to silence the science and practice of low-carbohydrate diets, motivated by a mixture of industry forces, institutional rigidities, longstanding biases and deeply entrenched interests – all of which are threatened by the success of a treatment that is the very opposite of what officials have espoused for decades.

Jennifer Elliott deregistered

The first sign in recent times that the practice of low-carb might be under attack came in 2015 out of New South Wales, Australia. The Dietitians Association of Australia (DAA) expelled dietician Jennifer Elliott, who after twenty years of recommending the standard low-fat, near-vegetarian diet, had shifted to a "lower carb" approach for her patients with obesity, diabetes, and other metabolic conditions. Elliott stumbled on this diet because while two of her children had thrived on the family regime of mostly grains, fruits and vegetables, her middle daughter, as a teen, grew nearly obese.[2] Elliott discovered that this daughter suffered from insulin resistance, and put her – successfully

– on a low-carb diet. These results along with an expanding knowledge of the science spurred Elliott not only to bring this approach to her practice but also to write a well-researched critique of the diet heart hypothesis, in *Food and Nutrition Sciences,* published in October, 2014.[3]

This article may have been what called Elliott to the attention of authorities. Soon thereafter, DAA began their proceedings against her and deregistered her, in May 2015, just five months later. DAA claimed that the reasons for its expulsion of Miss Elliott "DID NOT [sic] include the use of a low-carbohydrate diet." Instead, the group cited a number of seemingly trivial ways that Elliott's practice was allegedly substandard, such as "a lack of documented assessment of nutritional needs," and a failure to "demonstrate how your clinical assessment accounted for the patient's previous dietary knowledge,"[4] all of which pertain to Elliott's notes on a single client.[5] However, the DAA's stated reasons for expulsion also included the fact that Elliott made recommendations that are "inconsistent with Evidence-Based Practice." Thus, it seems that Elliott was indeed expelled, at least in part, for promoting the low-carb diet, which in Australia is not the standard of "evidence-based care."

Gary Fettke silenced

At the same time, the Australian Health Practitioners Regulation Agency (AHPRA) took up an anonymous complaint by a dietician in 2014 against Gary Fettke, an orthopaedic surgeon and senior lecturer at the University of Tasmania. The complaint alleged that he had, among other things, promoted "new ideas ... without substantial factual information" and claimed "inappropriately" to have "helped reverse Type 2 diabetes." In addition, by making speeches, AHPRA alleged that Fettke had the "potential to negatively impact on [sic] the lives of vulnerable, captive audiences."[6]

Fettke had discovered the low-carbohydrate diet around 2010 when he was overweight and pre-diabetic. The diet not only helped him with these conditions but also reversed an aggressive form of pituitary cancer with which he'd been diagnosed. Satisfied with the diet's efficacy as well as its evidence base, Fettke began to implement it among his diabetic patients, because one of the uglier ways that the disease manifests itself is in nerve damage and poor blood circulation, leading eventually to the need for amputation. As a surgeon, Fettke's job involved cutting off the toes, feet and limbs of these patients. Yet he found that by counseling them to restrict carbohydrates, this suffering could be avoided. Thus, in 2012, Fettke began to promote the low-carb diet publicly, on social media, at lectures, and on a popular website called "NoFructose.com."[7]

Rising prominence was again, a likely factor in triggering a response. APHRA, after conducting a closed-door investigation for two years and five months, issued a "caution"[8] against Fettke in November 2016, warning him "not [to] provide specific advice or recommendations on the subject of nutrition and how it relates to the management of diabetes or the treatment and/or prevention of cancer" because he was "not suitably trained or educated as a medical practitioner to be providing advice or recommendations on this topic."[9] While the complaint was irregular in quite a few ways, the point about training was simply illogical, because, as one doctor noted, Fettke had received the same amount of coursework on nutrition as anyone else in the Australian medical profession.[10]

APHRA's treatment of Fettke throughout the process was so unusual – in one instance demanding that he respond to a complex inquiry in less than an hour – that the Australian Senate launched an investigation into APHRA's overall handling of "vexatious complaints."* The Fettke episode alone comprised an entire chapter of the resulting 2017 report and included the finding that APHRA had indeed conducted itself in a number of ways that were highly questionable. The report states that the President of the Senate would therefore be enlisted to send a letter to all state agencies reminding them of the "need for care" in dealing with Senate witnesses such as Fettke.[11]

Nevertheless, Fettke remains banned for life from giving nutritional counseling to his patients or speaking out publicly on the subject.

The "Trial" of Tim Noakes

The events in Australia have been dwarfed by proceedings in South Africa, in what some have dubbed the "Nutrition Trial of the

---

* Defined by the Australian Senate as meaning those that are lodged primarily to bully or harass the practitioner subjected to it.

21st Century," In fact, it wasn't a trial but a hearing by the Health Professions Council of South Africa (HPSCA) over a single tweet by Professor Tim Noakes. This hearing, covered as front page news in South Africa and resounding around the world,[12, 13] has been by far the most high-profile example of efforts to punish and silence low-carb proponents.

Noakes is a world-famous exercise physiologist, now retired from the Division of Exercise and Sports Medicine at the University of Cape Town.[14] He is renowned for paradigm-changing breakthroughs in his field, including the revelation that athletes should not, actually, 'hydrate ahead of thirst,' as long thought. His various revelations have long ruffled the feathers of interested industries as well as his more traditional colleagues, yet these battles ultimately proved trivial compared to the nutrition debate into which Noakes inadvertently waded late in life.

When in his 60s, Noakes discovered that, despite being an accomplished marathoner, he was not only gaining weight but surprisingly, had contracted diabetes. Looking for a solution, he stumbled on a "New Atkins" diet book[15] and by following its advice, dramatically improved his health. Upon further investigations, Noakes came to the conclusion that, contrary to his longstanding "carb loading" recommendation, a high-carbohydrate diet was harmful not just for athletes but for anyone, like him, with insulin resistance. In a dramatic moment captured on a documentary film, Noakes recanted his previous position by opening a textbook on exercise he'd written and tearing out the pages on carb loading.[16]

After co-authoring a low-carb diet book called *The Real Meal Revolution* in 2013, Noakes become a virtual celebrity. (The book named low-carb the "Banting diet," after the Englishman William Banting who became famous in the 1870s upon discovering what he dubbed the "Banting" diet, or described simply as "to Bant.") Following publication of this run-away best-seller, Noakes could barely walk down the street without being recognised, often by people who had lost weight on his diet. "20 kilos, Professor!" they would call out to him, and, "Professor, 15 kilos and counting!"[17]

Yet Noakes was stunned and mortified to find that, due to his shifting views on nutrition, life-long colleagues turned against him. He lost the university lab that he had run for decades and was pushed into early retirement.[18] Nothing, however, could have prepared him for the ensuing years, spent embroiled in battling the South African authorities.

In early 2014, the Health Professionals Council of South Africa (HPCSA) responded to a formal complaint by Claire Julsing Strydom, then president of the Association for Dietetics in South Africa (ADSA), stating that that the "celebrity" Noakes had "inappropriately" tweeted "potentially life-threatening" low-carb advice to a breastfeeding mother. The tweet included the following: "Key is to ween [sic] baby onto LCHF" ("LCHF" refers to a diet low in carbohydrates and high in fat).

The HPCSA informed Noakes of the complaint shortly thereafter and nearly a full year later, decided to press charges against him. The HPCSA accused Noakes of being guilty of "unprofessional conduct...in that...you acted in a manner that is not in accordance with the norms and standards of your profession in that you provided unconventional advice on breastfeeding babies on social networks (tweet)."[19] At stake for Noakes was the loss of his medical license, a triviality, since he wasn't actively practising medicine, anyway. Instead, it was clear from the start that the issues on 'trial' were the low-carb diet and Noakes' professional reputation in promoting it.

The hearing unfolded over the next two years. A team of top lawyers volunteered to defend Noakes, and one expert witness flew in at her own expense.[20] Still, Noakes spent the equivalent of hundreds of thousands of dollars on the trial, including flying in three expert witnesses: dietician Caryn Zinn, Ph.D, the nutrition expert Zoë Harcombe, Ph.D, and me.[21] Our collective testimony covered key topics, including the fact that LCHF was actually consistent with current South African guidelines for infants, the lack of evidence to support the "conventional" advice and the far larger body of evidence supporting the "unconventional" advice.[22] Noakes' lawyers also argued that a mere exchange of tweets failed to establish the kind of doctor-patient relationship that would allow HPCSA jurisdiction to intervene in the first place. (Moreover, the HPCSA turned out to have no rules regarding the use of social media.)

A dramatic highlight of the hearing involved the publication of a 2014 paper,[23] by academics at a nearby university, which appeared to have been prepared specifically as evidence for the prosecution.[24] Indeed one of the paper's authors, Marjanne Senekal, sat with the prosecution team during a good part of the hearing. This, so-called "Naude *et al*" review found no advantage for the low-carb diet in the treatment of diabetes, and although this finding arguably ought to have been irrelevant for a case on infant weaning, it was nonetheless presented as a key piece of evidence against Noakes and incited a good deal of news coverage. A stunning blow to the paper came when, in her October 2016 testimony, Harcombe revealed that she and Noakes had a peer-reviewed critique in press, which documented "numerous errors, some material in nature" in the Naude paper, nearly all of which favored the prosecution's case.[25] The paper was thus critically undermined. (Naude and her team have not yet replied to the substantive issues of this critique, and as of this writing, the paper remains uncorrected.)[26]

On April 21, 2017, the HPCSA committee, in a 4-to-1 decision, found Noakes "not guilty." The ruling stated that the prosecution had not proven any harm from the tweet, that Noakes had not breached any norms or standards of the medical profession, and that his LCHF advice could not be found to be "not evidence based"[27] – which is to say that LCHF was in fact, evidence-based.

Noakes reacted with palpable relief, and in an interview, said, "It's been very, very demanding on us and on our lives and financially it's been huge. The real concern was the emotional strain that it had on us... As my wife said, did they ever consider the consequences for my wife and myself and our family? That was the hardest bit for both of us to cope with."[28]

Just weeks later, however, HPSCA filed an appeal, and a new panel will be selected to review the case again.[29]

Other tactics for silencing the science

In the cases above, health authorities can be seen as vehicles for repressing alternative scientific views. But what about those critics over whom these authorities have no jurisdiction? And what about renegade views that come not through people but via journal articles and books? Here, other tactics are used – and have long been used – to silence critics. It turns out that the field of nutrition science has a long and ugly history of bullying its dissenters, using a wide variety of unpleasant strategies.

One clear tactic has been to exclude and marginalise those scientists who break intellectual ranks. Over the last 50 years, critics of the diet-heart hypothesis have found that they've lost their research grants, been denied invitations to expert panels, and ceased to advance in the field. In my book, I describe a number of these cases in the U.S., including that of E. "Pete" Ahrens, a top lipid expert from the 1960s to the '90s at The Rockefeller University who, by the end of his career had trouble getting grants, because there was "a price to pay for going up against the establishment, and he was well aware of that," as a former student told me.[30] There was also George Mann, a biochemist who in the 1970s had been a director of the famed Framingham study, but because he persisted in challenging mainstream ideas about fat and cholesterol, lost his government research grant and found himself unable to publish his work. In the end, he was essentially expelled from his profession.[31]

In some cases, renegade scientists have been subject to actual harassment. For instance, several scientists who sounded the alarm on trans-fats in the 1970s, long before that issue went mainstream, found themselves attacked wherever they presented their work. In the audience at conferences were employees of the vegetable oil companies who worked as an organised group to protect trans-fats – their product – from any taint. They asked pointed questions during the question-and-answer period, intending to cast doubt on every aspect of challenging trans-fats research. One of those in the audience remembers going after Fred Kummerow, a prominent trans-fat critic: "We chased him at three or four conferences. Our objective was to sit in the audience, and when he stopped talking, to raise a lot of questions." Industry scientists would typically accuse research they didn't like as being "full of errors." "They would blindside you with something that was, in many cases, not even related to what you were saying," recalls Randall Wood, another trans-fat critic.[32] This treatment so dismayed Wood, in addition to stymieing his research, that he left his career as a scientist altogether. The impact of this harassment is clear: with the early trans-fats critics silenced and driven away, the health problems caused by these fats did not surface for another 20 years.

Occasionally, the harassment of researchers has taken a derisive turn into actual name-calling, although this practice seems to have been principally reserved for women. Biochemist Mary Enig, an early critic of trans-fats, was labeled by her colleagues as "nutso," "paranoid," "off-the-wall," and "a zealot."[33] And ever since I wrote "The Questionable Link Between Saturated Fat and Heart Disease," a top-emailed piece published in 2014 in the *Wall Street Journal*,[34] a researcher loosely associated with Yale University named David Katz has called me a series of names, including a "parasite of science,"[35] a "bully," a member of a "cabal,"[36] and "an animal unlike any I've ever seen before."[37]

Katz's attacks, though loathsome, are actually a compact study in the stratagems used to defend the status quo. In addition to name-calling, he often accuses anyone who disagrees with him of being motivated only by financial gain – for the sale of their books, for instance.[38] It is a hallmark of bias that these arguments are inconsistently applied, and are rarely, if ever, levied against scholars with books, even highly commercial diet books, that support establishment dogma.

Katz also tends to accuse diet-heart critics of being on the payroll of the meat or dairy industries. This is a long-standing technique going back to the 1970s, when the Chairman of the Food and Nutrition Board for the National Academy of Sciences, Al Harper, was attacked for getting funds from the meat industry. Harper and quite a few of his colleagues were at the time speaking out against the new low-fat dietary guidelines, about to be imposed by the US Department of Agriculture. Although nearly everyone on the Board had extensive ties to some part of the food industry, including the Hershey Food Corp. in one case, only ties to the meat industry were highlighted by the press.[39] This targeting of the meat industry above all others remains a bias in the US mainstream media. In 1980, *The New York Times*, a paper that has long promoted the low-fat diet, took the lead in pillorying Harper and ultimately sank his cautionary voice in the debate over the guidelines.[40]

This strategy of trying to link any diet-heart critic to the meat, dairy or egg industry has since been aggressively pursued by Center for Science in the Public Interest (CSPI), a long-time defender of the dietary guidelines. Any nutrition scientist or journalist who raises his or her voice to express doubts about the guidelines is attacked for links to these industries – meat, in particular.[41]

BMJ Retraction Effort and Dis-invitation

In researching my book, I was told an almost unbelievable story about how margarine executives in the 1970s had called up the editor of a scientific journal to try to prevent publication of an article that was critical of trans-fats. These executives were unsuccessful. But of course, once an article is published, the only way to suppress the science further is to demand retraction – which is precisely what happened to me, on an unprecedented scale, when I wrote a critical analysis of the expert report by the 2015 US HHS-USDA Dietary Guidelines advisory committee (DGAC), published in *The BMJ*.[42]

This analysis evaluated the entire body of science underpinning all the US Guidelines' key dietary recommendations and concluded that they were supported by "a miniscule quantity of rigorous evidence that only marginally supports claims that these diets can promote better health than alternatives." I found that the DGAC could identify only "limited" or "insufficient" evidence that the [USDA recommended] diets could combat diabetes and only "moderate" evidence that the diets can help people lose weight." I also found that the DGAC's finding that the evidence of a "strong" link between saturated fats and heart disease was not clearly supported by the evidence cited.

The article provoked an outrage among defenders of the guidelines. They submitted a number of criticisms through The BMJ's "rapid response" feature,[43, 44] which is the normal post-publication process, to which I responded.[45] Yet CSPI, unsatisfied with this process, wrote a letter demanding that The BMJ retract the article, based on a further 11 alleged errors. CSPI collected more than 180 signatures for its letter, from nutrition experts, graduate students and others around the world. Later it was revealed by *The Guardian* and bloggers in two countries that many of the letter signers knew nothing about the allegations in the letter they had signed; indeed, many had signed without asking a single question.[46] After more than a year of review, *The BMJ* announced that it would not retract the article, and *The BMJ* editor-in-chief Fiona Godlee wrote a strong commentary defending it and "its important critique of the advisory committee's processes for reviewing the evidence."[47]

This was certainly one of the biggest retraction efforts in the history of science, involving a policy that, more than any other, affects the world-wide epidemics of obesity and diabetes, yet the press barely covered it. Thus, another aspect of nutrition politics is revealed: the long-standing affinity of the press to status-quo dietary advice, which most news outlets have themselves been espousing for decades.

The U.S. press, as a separate, objective and critical actor in this field, has been virtually absent. (The U.K. press, by contrast, have been somewhat more independent.)

A final, classic example of how speech is effectively suppressed is through "dis-invitations" from events, which I also experienced. In early 2016, the Consumer Federation of America invited me to be on a panel at the National Food Policy Conference, a longstanding, major conference in Washington, D.C. I was to be the fourth member of a panel that also included the chair of the 2015 Dietary Guidelines Advisory Committee, the head of the Dietary Guidelines for the USDA, and the director of nutrition at the CSPI. However, the three other members of the panel threatened to quit if I were invited. So I was then disinvited.[48] A columnist for Spiked judged that my dis-invitation had been due to my critical views of the Dietary Guidelines and called it an "act of censorship."[49] Although one of my colleagues started a petition to reinstate me on the panel, which nearly 4,500 people signed in a week's time, I was not re-invited.[50]

Conclusion

Although my own role in the field obviously biases my approach to this material, the tactics described above – from name-calling to specious retraction efforts to the use of licensing boards to prosecute clearly vexatious complaints – appears to be a sustained, global effort to censor and silence alternative views of the science. The effect of these tactics extends far beyond the people who are immediately targeted. These people, including myself, have all clearly suffered, from stress to ourselves and our families, legal bills, the loss of colleagues, and diminished ability to act in the world. Yet these tactics are clearly meant to resound far beyond those of us who are directly targeted; the hearings and other attacks send a clear warning message to anyone who might even consider raising his or her voice in protest, and that message is: have no doubt, you will be pilloried, persecuted, and publicly vilified. Most people will not sign up for this. Thus the health establishment makes it clear to potential dissenters that the professional, personal, and financial risks of challenging the status-quo will be high.

To work in the field of nutrition science and to tolerate this kind of treatment of practitioners and researchers, whose crime is nothing

270

more than to challenge long-held beliefs about nutrition science based on their own observations or hard work, is to participate in an overtly shoddy set of standards for the field. One can legitimately ask, is it even a field of science? Science requires respectful dialogue and fair consideration of alternative ideas. Yet in nutrition we see the opposite: the systematic oppression and persecution of viewpoints that challenge the status-quo.

Certainly there are strong industry interests motivating these attacks. The sugar industry has been documented as a force behind the Noakes hearing,[51] and there are emerging suggestions of the same in the Fettke case. David Katz's motives are also likely to have been influenced by his vast ties to junk-food industries.[52] However, these motives cannot be disentangled from the tremendous incentive to preserve the status quo low-fat diet, endorsed by governments and professional associations around the world and which has been the foundation of every professional career in health and medical sciences for decades. To accept that this officially endorsed diet has harmed rather than helped people would clearly amount to a massive amount of cognitive dissonance that simply cannot be tolerated.

Thus, as evidence mounts for the superiority of a diet that is the exact opposite of this low-fat status quo, those who challenge the traditional advice and promote a low-carb diet for the management of obesity and diabetes can only expect ever-more heavy-handed and desperate attempts to shut down this science, along with its practitioners.

That is, until open and honest debate in the field of nutrition is allowed. It is beyond time for scientists to stand up for the principles of right and good science to make this happen.

Nina Teicholz

@bigfatsurprise
thebigfatsurprise.com
The Big Fat Surprise, Simon & Schuster 2014

Case Study: Neil

Cub leader Neil 'Baloo' Roberts was happily losing weight, but then realised why; he had late onset Type 1 diabetes. He followed official NHS advice until an unofficial pointer in a new direction changed his whole life. Now healthier and happier than ever, he says LCHF is the way to go for everyone.

My name is Neil Roberts, I am 49 years old and I'm a Cub Scout Leader in Derby, England. My pack name has always been 'Baloo', so if you can imagine a large, round, friendly bear, you can imagine that I was not a small person.

Back in February 2013, I was feeling rather pleased with myself. I had been counting calories in my 'healthy' low-fat diet, and was losing weight. In just a few weeks I had dropped from 12.5 stones (80 kg) to 11 stones (70 kg). At 5 ft 6" (168 cm), this took my BMI from 'almost obese' to 'normal'.

In real terms, that meant me smiling a lot, as people were commenting on how much better I looked.

All was not quite as rosy as it seemed though. I had been drinking

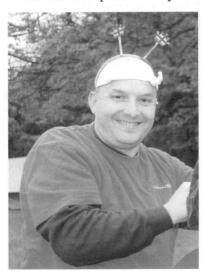

more and more liquid and urinating three times each night.

I distinctly remember drinking a pint of water, thinking it was the best drink ever, and drinking another straight away... and I was still thirsty an hour later. With memories of my father's late-onset Type 1 diabetes, I knew the symptoms, but I still put off going to see my GP... well, until my wife forced me.

I can still remember the nurse at the surgery talking to me as she took my blood glucose with a simple finger prick. It measured 13.3 mmol/L.

She went quiet, I just looked at her. She dodged my question about diabetes, and said further tests were needed.

I knew the answer, but was confused. I felt fine, I was even losing weight. How could I have diabetes?

I came out of denial soon. After all, there is a reason that the ancient Greeks called it the "melting disease": it's because you literally urinate your body tissues away. So that explained my weight loss!

I was hoping it was Type 2 diabetes, I felt I could somehow turn that around. Alas, no. Results showed that I was Type 1, and I was to carry on taking medications to try to keep my blood sugar down.

The diabetic clinic gave me the news that my pancreas was still producing some insulin, but that would stop within the year. I then had to look forward to sticking needles full of insulin into my belly.

The news didn't improve as I researched the disease: I was likely to die younger than most people; probably from a coronary episode.

I was not happy.

Then came the news that I absolutely must drastically reduce eating saturated fat, cheese, dairy, and red meats. I should only eat low-fat foods. The sheet of paper listed all the complex grains, heart healthy porridge oats, starchy foods I should eat; meals built around low GI carbohydrates and including plenty of fruit.

Oh joy.

Nevertheless, I knuckled under and decided I would be the best patient ever. I got my blood glucose down from a HbA1c of 10.1% to 6.8%. My health professionals thought this was good, and provided me syringes and insulin

My weight started to increase, but that didn't seem to matter, I was keeping low (ish) blood sugars.

Fast forward to October 2014, one and a half years since diagnosis. I was injecting 40 units of insulin a day and I thundered in at just over 13 stone (83.5 kg). That's a BMI of 29.6.

Baloo the fat Bear was back with a vengeance.

I tried and tried to lose weight, but it just wouldn't happen. My 'healthy' low-fat diet left me constantly hungry and the hypoglycemic blood sugar lows were awful.

On the bright side, my sugars weren't too bad and my cholesterol was nice and low. (Note: at that stage I was also taking statins like a good patient, but I'll leave the story of how better I feel without them for another book).

As October ticked over into November, everything changed.

I had a critical meeting with my diabetic nurse. She praised my numbers. Then, in passing, suggested I take a look at the work of a US doctor called Bernstein, and also consider slightly lowering my carbohydrate intake.

She just looked at me for a few seconds to make sure I had heard her. I was wondering why she was talking about my diet if my blood glucose levels weren't too bad? Yet I really felt she was trying to get something important across to me.

I was still pretty much following the NHS diet: I was eating 120 g – 200 g carbs per day; and injecting up to 40 units of insulin in total per day.

I experienced quite a few hypoglycaemic events, and was trying to control the peaks with quite a lot of insulin – injecting up to 40 units per day.

I'd invested in a Continuous Blood Glucose meter; one that is worn on your arm for two weeks at a time. It helped me work out how to keep my blood sugar from peaking above 7.8 mmol/L (140 mg/dL). I would try different doses and different times before and after meals.

One day I would almost manage it, the next it would fail. I was despondent.

I started to research more about the control of my blood sugar. From Harcombe and Cummins to Deakin and Noakes: I was transfixed. And Dr Bernstein's Diabetes Solution… well, what an epiphany!

The moment I finally realised that carbohydrate was the problem, not fat, then my life changed.

My Continuous Blood Glucose meter was exposing everything. I saw that eating mashed potato gave the same blood sugar response as eating candy floss. So I stopped eating them. Then I stopped bread, rice and pasta.

My blood glucose levels were looking fantastic.

I showed the results to my diabetic nurse, and she quietly admitted to eating a low-carb diet herself.

I learned a lot that day: that there was a reason she wasn't shouting about low-carb diets from the rooftops. It was not current health policy, so to advise it would have serious implications for her career.

For the record, I can honestly say that my (wonderful) diabetic nurse never, at any stage, advised me to switch to a low-carb diet.

I now eat a really healthy diet of high-fat (around 70%) low-carb food that my body actually needs.

Over the last few years, my facts and figures have been brilliant. I've maintained my current weight of 10 stone 5 pounds (66 kg) with a BMI of 23.4. I haven't needed an insulin injection in more than a year; in fact, I take no meds whatsoever.

What does that mean in real-terms? Well, my "Dad sleeps" after food are a thing of the past. I sleep better at night. I really enjoy my food.

And more than anything, I have FAR more energy. In fact, I often feel the need to cycle or break out into a run; it's like a fire inside. I remember this from when I was 20 years old.

And in our last race, Baloo outran all the Cubs when doing the athletes' badge.

On a serious note, I am now guiding all my friends, family (and anyone who will listen) into LCHF.

Ironically, it was my Type 1 diabetes that has improved my wife and children's health. They have reduced their sugar and carb intake dramatically. As has my mum...

She is 75 years old and has been a Type 2 diabetic for 15 years. Her LCHF lifestyle has dramatically improved her blood sugars (HbA1c 5.4% from 9%), and her weight is slowly dropping to a level she hasn't seen for decades.

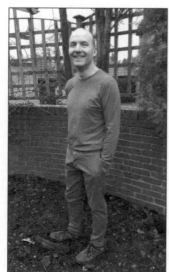

Reflecting on my experiences, I find I am upset that official NHS guidelines stop diabetics being told about LCHF immediately. I think that there is a glimmer of hope though.

Many staff in the NHS are clearly in the know, and if guidelines were to change, things could improve very quickly.

For my part, I have started talking to my local GP surgery about setting up a diabetes self-help group, with a focus on the benefits of a LCHF lifestyle. Initial indications are positive, and hopefully I can help spread the word and make a difference.

Baloo the thin bear.

References

All references were available at the time of publication.

Introduction

1 Banting W. *Corpulence: a letter addressed to the public.* Melbourne: W.B. Stephens, 1864.

2 Naude CE, Schoonees A, Senekal M, Young T, Garner P, Volmink J. Low Carbohydrate versus Isoenergetic Balanced Diets for Reducing Weight and Cardiovascular Risk: A Systematic Review and Meta-Analysis. PLoS One 2014.

3 https://therussells.crossfit.com/2017/01/05/big-food-vs-tim-noakes-the-final-crusade/

Chapter One

1. NCD Risk Factor Collaboration (NCD-RisC). Worldwide trends in diabetes since 1980: a pooled analysis of 751 population-based studies with 4.4 million participants. Lancet 2016.

2. Centers for Disease Control and Prevention. National diabetes statistics report: estimates of diabetes and its burden in the United States, 2014. Atlanta, GA: US Department of Health and Human Services, 2014.

3. Tuomilehto J. The emerging global epidemic of type 1 diabetes. Curr Diab Rep 2013; 13: 795–804.X.

4. International Diabetes Federation – A joint publication of the International Diabetes Federation and the International Working Group on the Diabetic Foot.

5. Morgan, C, J Peters, S Dixon, and C Currie. 2010. Estimates costs of acute hospital care for people with diabetes in the United Kingdom: a routine record linkage study in a large region. Diabetic Medicine 27:1066- 1073.

6. Kanavos P, van den Aardweg S, Schurer W (2012) Diabetes expenditure, burden of disease and management in 5 EU countries.

7. As reference 1.

8. As reference 6.

9. As reference 6.

10. Clarke, P , A Gray, R Legood, A Briggs, and R Holman. 2003. The impact of diabetes-related complications on healthcare costs: results from the United Kingdom Prospective Diabetes Study (UKPDS Study No. 65). Diabet Med. 20 (6):442-50.

11. As reference 1.

12. World Health Organisation – Global Report on Diabetes, 2016.

13. As reference 1.

14. Mainous et al. Prevalence of prediabetes in England from 2003 to 2011: population-based, cross- sectional study. BMJ Open 2014.

15. National Cardiovascular Intelligence Network (NCVIN). NHS Diabetes Prevention Programme (NHS DPP) Non-diabetic hyperglycemia. Public health England 2015.

16. International Diabetes Federation. IDF Diabetes Atlas, 7th edn, 2015. Brussels, Belgium.

17. Mozaffarian D et al. Lifestyle risk factors and new-onset diabetes mellitus in older adults: the cardiovascular health study. Arch Intern Med. 2009;169(8):798-807.

18. Ford ES et al. Healthy living is the best revenge. Arch Intern Med. 2009;169(15): 1355-62.

19. Edwardson C et al. Detection and early lifestyle intervention in those at risk of type 2 diabetes. EMJ Diabet. 2014;2:48-57.

20. Barry Eleanor, Roberts Samantha, Oke Jason, Vijayaraghavan Shanti, Normansell Rebecca, Greenhalgh Trisha et al. Efficacy and effectiveness of screen and treat policies in prevention of type 2 diabetes: systematic review and meta-analysis of screening tests and interventions BMJ 2017; 356 :i6538.

Chapter Two

1. Galassi, A et al. "Metabolic Syndrome and Risk of Cardiovascular Disease: A Meta-Analysis." The American Journal of Medicine. October 2006.

2. Howard Wolinsky. "Disease mongering and drug marketing." EMBO reports. July 2005.

3. http://www.diabetes.co.uk/diet/nhs-diet-advice.html

4. http://www.nhs.uk/Conditions/Diabetes-type2/Pages/Causes.aspx

5. http://www.diabetes.co.uk/diabetes-and-obesity.html

6. Gina Kolata. "Skinny and 119 pounds, but with the health hallmarks of obesity". NY Times. 22 July 2016.

Chapter Three

1. Pontiroli AE, Alberetto M, Pozza G. Patients with insulinoma show insulin resistance in the absence of arterial hypertension. Diabetologia. 1992 Mar; 35(3):294–5.

2. Pontiroli AE, Alberetto M, Capra F, Pozza G. The glucose clamp technique for the study of patients with hypoglycemia: insulin resistance as a feature of insulinoma. J Endocrinol Invest. 1990 Mar; 13(3):241–5.

3. Ghosh S et al. Clearance of acanthosis nigricans associated with insulinoma following surgical resection. QJM. 2008 Nov; 101(11):899–900. doi: 10.1093/qjmed/hcn098. Epub 2008 Jul 31. Accessed 8 April 2015.

4. Rizza RA et al. Production of insulin resistance by hyperinsulinemia in man. Diabetologia. 1985 Feb; 28(2):70–5.

5. Del Prato S et al. Effect of sustained physiologic hyperinsulinemia and hyperglycemia on insulin secretion and insulin sensitivity in man. Diabetologia. 1994 Oct; 37(10):1025–35.

6. Henry RR et al. Intensive Conventional Insulin Therapy for Type II Diabetes. Diabetes Care. 1993 Jan; 16(1):23–31.

7. Menke A et al. JAMA. 2015 Sep 8;314(10):1021-9. doi: 10.1001/jama.2015.10029. Prevalence of and Trends in Diabetes Among Adults in the United States, 1988-2012.

Chapter Four

1. World Health Organization: 2016: The ICD-10 Classification of Mental and Behavioural Disorders: Clinical descriptions and diagnostic guidelines.

2. Pressman P, Clemens RA, Rodriguez HA.Food Addiction: Clinical Reality or Mythology. Am J Med. 2015 Nov;128(11):1165-6.

3. US Senate Select Committee on Nutrition and Human Needs. Dietary Goals for the United States. 2nd edition. Washington (DC): US Government Printing Office, 1977.

4. Cywes, R. 1992 – Master of Science Thesis oral defense and Ph.D conversion – The influence and mechanism of hepatic reglycogenation on outcome of liver transplantation. Published 1995 – The role of platelets in hepatic allograft preservation-reperfusion injury. Doctoral Thesis. University of Toronto.

5. Obesityunderstood.com

6. Prochaska JO, Norcross JC, DiClemente CC. Changing for Good. Harper Collins. 2010.

7. Richards, JM. 2013 – MPH Thesis: Child/adolescent obesity and undiagnosed comorbidities: A case series study in bariatric medicine. University of North Florida.

8. Hopkins KF., DeCristofaro C, Elliott L. 2011. How can primary care providers manage pediatric obesity in the real world? Journal of the American Academy of Nurse Practitioners, 23(6), 278-288.

9. Standards of Medical Care in Diabetes—2013. Diabetes Care. 2013 Jan; 36(Suppl 1): S11–S66.

10. American Diabetes Association Diagnosis and classification of diabetes mellitus. Diabetes Care2010;33(Suppl. 1):S62–S69.

11. International Expert Committee report on the role of the A1C assay in the diagnosis of diabetes. Diabetes Care 2009;32:1327–1334.

12. Kapadia C, Zeitler P. Hemoglobin A1c measurement for the diagnosis of Type 2 diabetes in children; Drugs and Therapeutics Committee of the Pediatric Endocrine Society. Int J Pediatr Endocrinol. 2012 Dec 20;2012(1):31. doi: 10.1186/1687-9856-2012-31.

13. Zhang X, Gregg EW, Williamson DF, et al. A1C level and future risk of diabetes: a systematic review.Diabetes Care 2010;33:1665–1673.

14. Selvin E, Steffes MW, Zhu H, et al. Glycated hemoglobin, diabetes, and cardiovascular risk in nondiabetic adults. N Engl J Med 2010;362:800–811.

15. Zhang X, Gregg EW, Williamson DF, et al. A1C level and future risk of diabetes: a systematic review.Diabetes Care 2010;33:1665–1673.

16. Goh YM, Toumi Z, Date RS. Surgical cure for type 2 diabetes by foregut or hindgut operations: a myth or reality? A systematic review. Surg Endosc. 2016 May 18.

Chapter Five

1. Richard Bernstein, *Dr Bernstein's Diabetes Solution: A Complete Guide to Achieving Normal Blood Sugars*. 4th revised edition. Published by Little Brown. December 2011

2. Feinman RD, Pogozelski WK, Astrup A, et al. Dietary Carbohydrate restriction as the first approach in diabetes management. Critical review and evidence base. Nutrition (Burbank, Los Angeles County, Calif.) 2014.

3. http://nutritiondata.self.com/facts/fats-and-oils/508/2

4. http://nutritiondata.self.com/facts/dairy-and-egg-products/133/2

Chapter Six

1. Dagens Medicin (Today's Pharmacy). 7th April 2009. by Simon Rothelius with Dr Uffe Ravnskov.

https://www.dagensmedicin.se/artiklar/2009/04/07/livsmedelsverket-bor-omedelbart-sluta-med-kostrad-till-allmanheten/

2. "Om behandlingen av sockersjuka (även med insulin)", by Karl Petrén. 1926. Publisher: Uppsala, Almqvist & Wiksell. (https://www.ncbi.nlm.nih.gov/nlmcatalog/188922).

Chapter Eight

1. Petrisor B, Bhandari M. The hierarchy of evidence: Levels and grades of recommendation. Indian J Orthop. 2007;41:11-5. doi: 10.4103/0019-5413.30519.

2. Taubes G. Good Calories, Bad Calories. New York City, New York, United States: Alfred A. Knopf; 2007.

3. Teicholz N. The Big Fat Surprise: Why Butter, Meat and Cheese Belong in a Healthy Diet. New York City, New York, United States: Simon and Schuster; 2014.

4. Crofts C, Zinn C, Wheldon M, Schofield G. Hyperinsulinemia: A unifying theory of chronic disease? Diabesity. 2015;1:34-43. doi:

5. Kraft J. Diabetes Epidemic & You. Bloomington, Indiana, United States: Trafford Publishing 2008.

6. Crofts C, Schofield G, Zinn C, Wheldon M, Kraft J. Identifying hyperinsulinaemia in the absence of impaired glucose tolerance: An examination of the Kraft database. Diabetes Res Clin Pract. 2016;118:50-7. doi: 10.1016/j.diabres.2016.06.007.

7. Dietitians NZ. Nutritional Management of Type 2 Diabetes Mellitus: Dietitians New Zealand Diabetes Dietitian Special Interest Group.; 2015.

8. Schofield G, Zinn C, Rodger C. What The Fat? Fat's in Sugar's out. Auckland, New Zealand: The Real Food Publishing Company; 2015.

Chapter Nine

1. Marathe PH, Gao HX, Close KL. American Diabetes Association Standards of Medical Care in Diabetes 2017. Journal of diabetes. 2017. Epub 2017/01/11.

2. Khaw KT, Wareham N, Luben R, Bingham S, Oakes S, Welch A, et al. Glycated haemoglobin, diabetes, and mortality in men in Norfolk cohort of european prospective investigation of cancer and nutrition (EPIC-Norfolk). BMJ. 2001;322(7277):15-8. Epub 2001/01/05.

3. Khaw KT, Wareham N, Bingham S, Luben R, Welch A, Day N. Association of hemoglobin A1c with cardiovascular disease and mortality in adults: the European prospective investigation into cancer in Norfolk. Ann Intern Med. 2004;141(6):413-20. Epub 2004/09/24.

4. Selvin E, Coresh J, Golden SH, Brancati FL, Folsom AR, Steffes MW. Glycemic control and coronary heart disease risk in persons with and without diabetes: the atherosclerosis risk in communities study. Archives of internal medicine. 2005;165(16):1910-6. Epub 2005/09/15.

5. Barr EL, Boyko EJ, Zimmet PZ, Wolfe R, Tonkin AM, Shaw JE. Continuous relationships between non-diabetic hyperglycemia and both cardiovascular disease and all-cause mortality: the Australian Diabetes, Obesity, and Lifestyle (AusDiab) study. Diabetologia. 2009;52(3):415-24. Epub 2009/01/09.

6. Garg N, Moorthy N, Kapoor A, Tewari S, Kumar S, Sinha A, et al. Hemoglobin a1c in nondiabetic patients: an independent predictor of coronary artery disease and its severity. Mayo Clinic proceedings Mayo Clinic. 2014;89(7):908-16. Epub 2014/07/06.

7. Bernstein RK. Dr Bernstein's Diabetes Solution: INGP; 2011. 544 p.

8. Rasmussen OW, Gregersen S, Dorup J, Hermansen K. Blood glucose and insulin responses to different meals in non-insulin-dependent diabetic subjects of both sexes. The American journal of clinical nutrition. 1992;56(4):712-5. Epub 1992/10/01.

Chapter Ten

1. Atkinson, F. S., Foster-Powell, K., et al. (2008). "International tables of glycemic index and glycemic load values: 2008." Diabetes Care 31(12): 2281-2283.

2. Unwin D, Unwin J. Low carbohydrate diet to achieve weight loss and improve HbA1c in type 2 diabetes and pre-diabetes: experience from one general practice. Practical Diabetes 2014;31(2):76-79 doi: 10.1002/pdi.1835.

3. Anstee QM, McPherson S, Day CP. How big a problem is non-alcoholic fatty liver disease? Bmj 2011;343:d3897.

4. Douglas S. Lee, Jane C. Evans, Sander J. Robins. Gamma Glutamyl Transferase and Metabolic Syndrome, Cardiovascular Disease, and Mortality Risk.The Framingham Heart Study.Arteriosclerosis, Thrombosis, and Vascular Biology. 2007; 27: 127-133.

5. Raised GGT levels, Diabetes and NAFLD: Is dietary carbohydrate a link? Primary care pilot of a low carbohydrate diet. David J. Unwin, Daniel J. Cuthbertson, Richard Feinman & Victoria S. Sprung. Diabesity in Practice; September 2015.

6. Taylor R. The 2012 Banting Lecture. Reversing the twin cycles of Type 2 diabetes. Diabetic medicine : a journal of the British Diabetic Association 2012.

7. Fraser A, Harris R, Sattar N, et al. Alanine aminotransferase, gamma-glutamyltransferase, and incident diabetes: the British Women's Heart and Health Study and meta-analysis. Diabetes Care 2009;32(4):741-50.

8. Marchesini G, Avagnina S, Barantani EG, et al. Aminotransferase and gamma-glutamyltranspeptidase levels in obesity are associated with insulin resistance and the metabolic syndrome. J Endocrinol Invest 2005;28(4):333-9.

9. As reference 5.

10. Unwin D, Haslam D, Livesey G. It is the glycaemic response to, not the carbohydrate content of food that matters in diabetes and obesity: The glycaemic index revisited. Journal of Insulin Resistance 2016;1(1).

Chapter Eleven

1. Bradford Hill A. The Environment and Disease: Association or Causation? Proc. R. Soc. Med. 1965;58(5):295-300

2. Harcombe Z. Dietary fat guidelines have no evidence base: where next for public health nutritional advice? Br. J. Sports Med. 2016 doi: 10.1136/bjsports-2016-096734[published Online First: Epub Date].

3. Keys A. Coronary heart disease in seven countries I. The study program and objectives. Circulation 1970;41(I-1-I-8) doi: 10.1161/01.CIR.41.4S1.I-1 [published Online First: Epub Date].

4. Stuckey NW. Uber die Veranderungen der kaninchen aorta bei der reichlichen tierischen kost. Zentralbl. Allg. Pathol. Pathol. Anat. 1910;21:668

5. Stuckey NW. Uber die Veranderungen der kaninchen aorta unter der Wirkung reichlicher tierscher nahrung. Zentralbl. Allg. Pathol. Pathol. Anat. 1911;22:379-80

6. Stuckey NW. Uber die Veranderungen der kaninchen-aorta bei der futterung mit verschiedenen fettsorten. Zentralbl. Allg. Pathol. Pathol. Anat. 1912;23:910-11

7. Chalatow SS. Uber das verhalten der leber gegenuber den verschiedenen arten von Speisefett. Virchows Arch. Pathol. Anat. Physiol. Klin. Med. 1912;**207**:452-69

8. Wesselkin NW. Uber die Ablagerung von fettartigen Stoffen in den Organen. Virchows Arch. Pathol. Anat. Physiol. Klin. Med. 1913;**212**:225-35

9. Anitschkow N. Über die Veränderungen der Kaninchenaorta bei experimenteller Cholesterinsteatose. Beitr Pathol Anat. 1913;**56**:379-404

10. Kon Y. Referat uber arteriosklerose. Trans. Jpn. Pathol. Soc. 1913;**3**:8-19

11. Kon Y. Futterungsversuche an Saugetieren mit leberpulver und eigelb. Trans. Jpn. Pathol. Soc. 1914;**4**:105-12

12. Knack AV. Uber cholesterinsklerose. Virchows Arch. Pathol. Anat. Physiol. Klin. Med. 1915;**220**:36-52

13. Keys A, Anderson JT. The relationship of the diet to the development of atherosclerosis in man. In: National Research Council DoMS, ed. Symposium on atherosclerosis. Washington: National Academy of Sciences – National Research Council., 1954:181-96.

14. Keys A, Mickelsen O, Miller EvO, Chapman CB. The Relation in Man between Cholesterol Levels in the Diet and in the Blood. Science (New York, N.Y.) 1950;**112**(2899):79-81 doi: 10.1126/science.112.2899.79 [published Online First: Epub Date].

15. Keys A. Human atherosclerosis and the diet. Circulation 1952;**5**(1):115-8

16. Keys A. The cholesterol problem. Voeding 1952;**13**:539-55

17. Keys A. The diet and the development of coronary heart disease. J. Chronic Dis. 1956;**4**(4):364-80

18. Keys A, Fidanza F, Scardi V, Bergami G, Keys MH, di Lorenzo F. Studies on serum cholesterol and other characteristics of clinically healthy men in Naples. Arch. Int. Med., 1954;**93**:328-36

19. Keys A. Atherosclerosis: a problem in newer public health. J. Mt. Sinai Hosp. N. Y. 1953;**20**(2):118-39

20. Yerushalmy J, Hilleboe HE. Fat in the diet and mortality from heart disease; a methodologic note. N. Y. State J. Med. 1957;**57**(14):2343-54

21. Bronte-Stewart B, Keys A, Brock JF. Serum-Cholesterol, diet and coronary heart-disease: An inter-racial survey in the Cape Peninsula. The Lancet 1955;**266**(6900):1103-08 doi: http://dx.doi.org/10.1016/S0140-6736(55)92947-0 [published Online First: Epub Date].

22. Keys A. Diet and the epidemiology of coronary heart disease. J. Am. Med. Assoc. 1957;**164**(17):1912-19 doi: 10.1001/jama.1957.62980170024007e [published Online First: Epub Date].

23. Harcombe Z, Baker JS, Cooper SM, et al. Evidence from randomised controlled trials did not support the introduction of dietary fat guidelines in 1977 and 1983: a systematic review and meta-analysis. Open Heart 2015;**2**(1) doi: 10.1136/openhrt-2014-000196 [published Online First: Epub Date].

24. Harcombe Z, Baker JS, Davies B. Evidence from prospective cohort studies did not support the introduction of dietary fat guidelines in 1977 and 1983: a systematic review. Br. J. Sports Med. 2016 doi: 10.1136/bjsports-2016-096409 [published Online First: Epub Date].

25. Harcombe Z, Baker JS, DiNicolantonio JJ, Grace F, Davies B. Evidence from randomised controlled trials does not support current dietary fat guidelines: a systematic review and meta-analysis. Open Heart 2016;3(2) doi: 10.1136/openhrt-2016-000409 [published Online First: Epub Date].

26. Harcombe Z, Baker J, Davies B. Evidence from prospective cohort studies does not support current dietary fat guidelines: A systematic review and meta-analysis. Br. J. Sports Med. 2016 doi: doi:10.1136/bjsports-2016-096550 [published Online First: Epub Date].

27. Watts GF, Lewis B, Brunt JN, et al. Effects on coronary artery disease of lipid-lowering diet, or diet plus cholestyramine, in the St Thomas' Atherosclerosis Regression Study (STARS). The Lancet 1992;339(8793):563-9

28. Burr ML, Fehily AM, Gilbert JF, et al. Effects of changes in fat, fish, and fibre intakes on death and myocardial reinfarction: diet and reinfarction trial (DART). The Lancet 1989;2(8666):757-61

29. Research Committee. Low-fat diet in myocardial infarction: A controlled trial. The Lancet 1965;2(7411):501-4

30. Howard BV, Van Horn L, Hsia J, et al. Low-fat dietary pattern and risk of cardiovascular disease: the Women's Health Initiative Randomized Controlled Dietary Modification Trial. JAMA 2006;295(6):655-66 doi: 10.1001/jama.295.6.655 [published Online First: Epub Date].

31. Woodhill JM, Palmer AJ, Leelarthaepin B, McGilchrist C, Blacket RB. Low fat, low cholesterol diet in secondary prevention of coronary heart disease. Advances in experimental medicine and biology 1978;109:317-30

32. Frantz ID, Dawson EA, Ashman PL, et al. Test of effect of lipid lowering by diet on cardiovascular risk. The Minnesota Coronary Survey. Arteriosclerosis, Thrombosis, and Vascular Biology 1989;9(1):129-35 doi: 10.1161/01.atv.9.1.129 [published Online First: Epub Date].

33. Keys A. Coronary heart disease in seven countries Summary. Circulation 1970;41(I-186-I-195) doi: 10.1161/01.CIR.41.4S1.I-186 [published Online First: Epub Date].

34. Boniface DR, Tefft ME. Dietary fats and 16-year coronary heart disease mortality in a cohort of men and women in Great Britain. Eur. J. Clin. Nutr. 2002;56(8):786-92 doi: 10.1038/sj.ejcn.1601509 [published Online First: Epub Date].

35. Xu J, Eilat-Adar S, Loria C, et al. Dietary fat intake and risk of coronary heart disease: the Strong Heart Study. The American journal of clinical nutrition 2006;84(4):894-902

36. Rose GA, Thomson WB, Williams RT. Corn Oil in Treatment of Ischaemic Heart Disease. BMJ 1965;1(5449):1531-33 doi: 10.1136/bmj.1.5449.1531 [published Online First: Epub Date].

37. Dayton S, Pearce ML, Hashomoto S, Dixon WJ, Tomiyasu U. A Controlled Clinical Trial of a Diet High in Unsaturated Fat in Preventing Complications of Atherosclerosis. Circulation 1969;**40**(1S2):II-1-II-63 doi: 10.1161/01.cir.40.1s2.ii-1 [published Online First: Epub Date].

38. European Medicines Agency. Repatha INN-evolocumab: Summary of Product Characteristics,. In: Agency EM, ed. June 2015 ed, 2015:71.

39. Ostlund RE, Jr. Phytosterols in human nutrition. Annu. Rev. Nutr. 2002;**22**:533-49 doi: 10.1146/annurev.nutr.22.020702.075220 [published Online First: Epub Date].

40. Weihrauch JL, Gardner JM. Sterol content of foods of plant origin. Journal of the American Dietetic Association 1978;**73**(1):39-47

41. Pollak OJ. Reduction of Blood Cholesterol in Man. Circulation 1953;**7**(5):702-06 doi: 10.1161/01.cir.7.5.702[published Online First: Epub Date].

42. Harcombe Z, Baker J. Plant Sterols lower cholesterol, but increase risk for Coronary Heart Disease. Online J. Biol. Sci. 2014;**14**(3):167-69 doi: 10.3844/ojbssp.2014.167.169 [published Online First: Epub Date].

43. Esrey KL, Joseph L, Grover SA. Relationship between dietary intake and coronary heart disease mortality: Lipid Research Clinics Prevalence Follow-Up Study. J. Clin. Epidemiol. 1996;**49**(2):211-16 doi: http://dx.doi.org/10.1016/0895-4356(95)00066-6 [published Online First: Epub Date].

44. Willett WC. Nutritional epidemiology issues in chronic disease at the turn of the century. Epidemiol. Rev. 2000;**22**(1):82-6

45. Cook A, Pryer J, Shetty P. The problem of accuracy in dietary surveys. Analysis of the over 65 UK National Diet and Nutrition Survey. J. Epidemiol. Community Health 2000;**54**(8):611-16 doi: 10.1136/jech.54.8.611 [published Online First: Epub Date].

46. Kipnis V, Midthune D, Freedman L, et al. Empirical evidence of correlated biases in dietary assessment instruments and its implications. Am. J. Epidemiol. 2001;**153**:394 – 403

47. Archer E, Pavela G, Lavie CJ. The Inadmissibility of What We Eat in America and NHANES Dietary Data in Nutrition and Obesity Research and the Scientific Formulation of National Dietary Guidelines. Mayo Clin. Proc. 2015;**90**(7):911-26 doi: 10.1016/j.mayocp.2015.04.009 [published Online First: Epub Date].

48. Beaton GH, Milner J, McGuire V, Feather TE, Little JA. Source of variance in 24-hour dietary recall data: implications for nutrition study design and interpretation. Carbohydrate sources, vitamins, and minerals. The American journal of clinical nutrition 1983;**37**(6):986-95

49. Freedman LS, Schatzkin A, Wax Y. The impact of dietary measurement error on planning sample size required in a cohort study. Am. J. Epidemiol. 1990;**132**(6):1185-95

50. Keys A. Coronary heart disease in seven countries XVII. The Diet Circulation 1970;**41**(I-162-I-183) doi: 10.1161/01.CIR.41.4S1.I-162 [published Online First: Epub Date].

51. Personal communication. Personal meeting with Professor Peter Elwood, 14 August 2015. Cardiff, 2015.

52. Yudkin J. Diet and coronary thrombosis: Hypothesis and fact. The Lancet 1957;**270**(6987):155-62

53. Mente A, de Koning L, Shannon HS, Anand SS. A systematic review of the evidence supporting a causal link between dietary factors and coronary heart disease. Arch. Intern. Med. 2009;**169**(7):659-69 doi: 10.1001/archinternmed.2009.38 [published Online First: Epub Date].

54. Select Committee on Nutrition and Human Needs. *Dietary goals for the United States*. First ed. Washington: U.S. Govt. Print. Off., February 1977.

55. National Advisory Committee on Nutritional Education (NACNE). A discussion paper on proposals for nutritional guidelines for health education in Britain. London: The Health Education Council, 1983.

56. Select committee on nutrition and human needs. *Dietary goals for the United States, supplemental views*. Washington: U.S. Govt. Print. Off., 1977.

57. Ancel Keys P. Front Cover. Time Magazine, Jan 13 1961:Vol. LXXVII No.3.

58. Schwingshackl L, Hoffmann G. Dietary fatty acids in the secondary prevention of coronary heart disease: a systematic review, meta-analysis and meta-regression. BMJ Open 2014;**4**(4) doi: 10.1136/bmjopen-2013-004487 [published Online First: Epub Date].

59. Hooper L, Summerbell CD, Thompson R, et al. Reduced or modified dietary fat for preventing cardiovascular disease. Cochrane database of systematic reviews (Online) 2011(7):CD002137 doi: 10.1002/14651858.CD002137.pub2 [published Online First: Epub Date].

60. Mozaffarian D, Micha R, Wallace S. Effects on coronary heart disease of increasing polyunsaturated fat in place of saturated fat: a systematic review and meta-analysis of randomized controlled trials. PLoS Med. 2010;**7**:e1000252

61. Hooper L, Martin N, Abdelhamid A, Davey Smith G. Reduction in saturated fat intake for cardiovascular disease. Cochrane Database of Systematic Reviews 2015(6) doi: 10.1002/14651858.CD011737 [published Online First: Epub Date].

62. Siri-Tarino PW, Sun Q, Hu FB, Krauss RM. Meta-analysis of prospective cohort studies evaluating the association of saturated fat with cardiovascular disease. The American journal of clinical nutrition 2010;**91**(3):535-46 doi: 10.3945/ajcn.2009.27725 [published Online First: Epub Date].

63. Skeaff CM, Miller J. Dietary fat and coronary heart disease: summary of evidence from prospective cohort and randomised controlled trials. Ann. Nutr. Metab. 2009;**55**(1-3):173-201 doi: 10.1159/000229002 [published Online First: Epub Date].

64. Chowdhury R, Warnakula S, Kunutsor S, et al. Association of Dietary, Circulating, and Supplement Fatty Acids With Coronary Risk: A Systematic Review and Meta-analysis. Ann. Intern. Med. 2014;**160**(6):398-406 doi: 10.7326/M13-1788 [published Online First: Epub Date].

65. Ravnskov U, DiNicolantonio JJ, Harcombe Z, Kummerow FA, Okuyama H, Worm N. The Questionable Benefits of Exchanging Saturated Fat With Polyunsaturated Fat. Mayo Clinic proceedings. Mayo Clinic 2014

66. Turpeinen O, Karvonen MJ, Pekkarinen M, Miettinen M, Elosuo R, Paavilainen E. Dietary prevention of coronary heart disease: the Finnish Mental Hospital Study. Int J Epidemiol 1979;**8**(2):99-118

67. Miettinen M, Turpeinen O, Karvonen MJ, Pekkarinen M, Paavilainen E, Elosuo R. Dietary prevention of coronary heart disease in women: the Finnish mental hospital study. Int J Epidemiol 1983;**12**(1):17-25

68. Houtsmuller AJ, Zahn KJ, Henkes HE. Unsaturated fats and progression of diabetic retinopathy. Doc. Ophthalmol. 1979;**48**(2):363-71 doi: 10.1007/BF00141465 [published Online First: Epub Date].

69. Black HS, Herd JA, Goldberg LH, et al. Effect of a Low-Fat Diet on the Incidence of Actinic Keratosis. New England Journal of Medicine 1994;**330**(18):1272-75 doi: doi:10.1056/NEJM199405053301804 [published Online First: Epub Date].

70. Moy TF, Yanek LR, Raqueño JV, et al. Dietary Counseling for High Blood Cholesterol in Families at Risk of Coronary Disease. Prev. Cardiol. 2001;**4**(4):158-64 doi: 10.1111/j.1520-037X.2001.00543.x [published Online First: Epub Date].

71. Ley SJ, Metcalf PA, Scragg RK, Swinburn BA. Long-term effects of a reduced fat diet intervention on cardiovascular disease risk factors in individuals with glucose intolerance. Diabetes Res. Clin. Pract. 2004;**63**(2):103-12

72. Select Committee on Nutrition and Human Needs. *Dietary goals for the United States*. Second ed. Washington: U.S. Govt. Print. Off., December 1977.

73. Harcombe Z, Baker J, Davies B. Food for Thought: Have We Been Giving the Wrong Dietary Advice? Food and Nutrition Sciences 2013;**4**(3):240-44 doi: 10.4236/fns.2013.43032 [published Online First: Epub Date].

74. Tanner TH. *The Practice of Medicine*. Philadelphia: Lindsay & Blakiston, 1869.

75. Centers for Disease Control and Prevention. Table 71. Overweight, obesity, and healthy weight among persons 20 years of age and over, by selected characteristics: United States, selected years 1960-1962 through 2005-2008,. In: National Center for Health Statistics, ed., 2010.

76. Michael Wadsworth, Diana Kuh, Marcus Richards, Hardy. R. Cohort Profile: The 1946 National Birth Cohort (MRC National Survey of Health and Development). Int J Epidemiol 2006;**35**:49-54 doi: 10.1093/ije/dyi201 [published Online First: Epub Date].

77. Centers for Disease Control and Prevention. Long term trends in diabetes. In: Translation CDoD, ed.: Centers for Disease Control and Prevention, October 2014.

78. Department of Health and Human Services (HHS). Dietary Guidelines for Americans. In: Department of Health and Human Services (HHS), ed., 2010.

79. Centers for Disease Control and Prevention. National diabetes statistics report: estimates of diabetes and its burden in the United States,: U.S. Department of Health and Human Services, 2014.

80. Gregg EW, Zhuo X, Cheng YJ, Albright AL, Narayan KMV, Thompson TJ. Trends in lifetime risk and years of life lost due to diabetes in the USA, 1985-2011: a modelling study. The Lancet Diabetes & Endocrinology 2014

81. Diabetes UK. Diabetes in the UK 2004: A report from Diabetes UK October 2004. Available at www.diabetes.org.uk/Documents/Reports/in_the_UK_2004.doc, 2004:27.

82. Diabetes UK. Diabetes: Facts and stats. Available at https://www.diabetes.org. uk/Documents/Position%20statements/Facts%20and%20stats%20June%202015. pdf, 2015:22.

83. Lawrence GD. Dietary Fats and Health: Dietary Recommendations in the Context of Scientific Evidence. Advances in Nutrition: An International Review Journal 2013;4(3):294-302 doi: 10.3945/an.113.003657 [published Online First: Epub Date].

84. Malhotra A. Saturated fat is not the major issue. BMJ 2013;347 doi: 10.1136/bmj. f6340 [published Online First: Epub Date].

85. DiNicolantonio JJ. The cardiometabolic consequences of replacing saturated fats with carbohydrates or Ω-6 polyunsaturated fats: Do the dietary guidelines have it wrong? Open Heart 2014;1(1) doi: 10.1136/openhrt-2013-000032 [published Online First: Epub Date].

86. Hansen A. Swedish health advisory body says too much carbohydrate, not fat, leads to obesity. BMJ 2013;347 doi: 10.1136/bmj.f6873 [published Online First: Epub Date].

87. Feinman RD, Pogozelski WK, Astrup A, et al. Dietary Carbohydrate restriction as the first approach in diabetes management. Critical review and evidence base. Nutrition (Burbank, Los Angeles County, Calif.) 2014

88. Dietary Guidelines Advisory Committee. Scientific Report of the 2015 Dietary Guidelines Advisory Committee. In: Department of Health and Human Services (HHS), ed., 2015:571.

89. Committee on Medical Aspects of Food Policy (COMA). Diet and cardiovascular disease: Report of the panel on diet in relation to cardiovascular disease, 1984.

90. Department of Health. Dietary Reference Values for Food Energy and Nutrients for the United Kingdom,. In: Department of Health, ed. Report of the Panel on Dietary Reference Values of the Committee on Medical Aspects of Food Policy: The Stationery Office, 1991:212.

91. Schwab U, Uusitupa M. Diet heart controversies – Quality of fat matters. Nutrition, Metabolism and Cardiovascular Diseases 2015;25(7):617-22 doi: http://dx.doi. org/10.1016/j.numecd.2015.03.009 [published Online First: Epub Date].

92. Li Y, Hruby A, Bernstein AM, et al. Saturated Fats Compared With Unsaturated Fats and Sources of Carbohydrates in Relation to Risk of Coronary Heart Disease: A Prospective Cohort Study. J. Am. Coll. Cardiol. 2015;66(14):1538-48 doi: 10.1016/j. jacc.2015.07.055 [published Online First: Epub Date].

93. Jakobsen MU, O'Reilly EJ, Heitmann BL, et al. Major types of dietary fat and risk of coronary heart disease: a pooled analysis of 11 cohort studies. The American journal of clinical nutrition 2009;**89**(5):1425-32 doi: 10.3945/ajcn.2008.27124 [published Online First: Epub Date].

94. de Souza RJ, Mente A, Maroleanu A, et al. Intake of saturated and trans unsaturated fatty acids and risk of all cause mortality, cardiovascular disease, and type 2 diabetes: systematic review and meta-analysis of observational studies. BMJ 2015;**351** doi: 10.1136/bmj.h3978 [published Online First: Epub Date].

95. Lamarche B, Couture P. It is time to revisit current dietary recommendations for saturated fat. Applied Physiology, Nutrition, and Metabolism 2014:1-3 doi: 10.1139/apnm-2014-0141 [published Online First: Epub Date].

96. Ramsden CE, Hibbeln JR, Majchrzak SF, Davis JM. n-6 Fatty acid-specific and mixed polyunsaturate dietary interventions have different effects on CHD risk: a meta-analysis of randomised controlled trials. British Journal of Nutrition 2010;**104**(11):1586-600 doi: doi:10.1017/S0007114510004010 [published Online First: Epub Date].

97. Ramsden CE, Zamora D, Leelarthaepin B, et al. Use of dietary linoleic acid for secondary prevention of coronary heart disease and death: evaluation of recovered data from the Sydney Diet Heart Study and updated meta-analysis. BMJ 2013;**346** doi: 10.1136/bmj.e8707 [published Online First: Epub Date].

98. Baum SJ, Kris-Etherton PM, Willett WC, et al. Fatty acids in cardiovascular health and disease: a comprehensive update. Journal of clinical lipidology 2012;**6**(3):216-34 doi: 10.1016/j.jacl.2012.04.077 [published Online First: Epub Date].

99. Burr ML, Ashfield-Watt PAL, Dunstan FDJ, et al. Lack of benefit of dietary advice to men with angina: results of a controlled trial. Eur. J. Clin. Nutr. 2003;**57**(2):193-200

100. Schmitz G, Ecker J. The opposing effects of n−3 and n−6 fatty acids. Prog. Lipid Res. 2008;**47**(2):147-55 doi: http://dx.doi.org/10.1016/j.plipres.2007.12.004 [published Online First: Epub Date].

101. A National Statistics Publication. The Family Food Survey. In: DEFRA, ed.: The Department for Environment, Food and Rural Affairs, 2010.

102. Gowlett JAJ. What Actually was the Stone Age Diet? Journal of Nutritional and Environmental Medicine 2003;**13**(3):143-47 doi: 10.1080/13590840310001619338 [published Online First: Epub Date].

103. CBS News. Exchange between Dr Robert Olson and Senator George McGovern from The United States Senate Select Committee on Nutrition and Human Needs. Washington, July 26 1977.

104. Stegemann C, Pechlaner R, Willeit P, et al. Lipidomics profiling and risk of cardiovascular disease in the prospective population-based Bruneck study. Circulation 2014;**129**(18):1821-31 doi: 10.1161/circulationaha.113.002500 [published Online First: Epub Date].

Chapter Twelve

1. Windaus A. Uber der Gehalt normaler und atheromatöser Aorten an Cholesterol und Cholesterinester. Zeitschrift Physiol Chemie. 1910;67:174-76.

2. Anitschkow N. Über die Veränderungen der Kaninchenaorta bei experimenteller Cholesterinsteatose. Beitr Pathol Anat. 1913;56:379-404.

3. Gofman JW, Lindgren F. The role of lipids and lipoproteins in atherosclerosis. Science (New York, N.Y.) 1950;111(2877):166-71.

4. Keys A. Coronary heart disease in seven countries I. The study program and objectives. Circulation 1970;41(I-1-I-8) doi: 10.1161/01.CIR.41.4S1.I-1.

5. Keys A. Seven countries: a multivariate analysis of death and coronary heart disease: Harvard University Press, 1980.

6. Select Committee on Nutrition and Human Needs. Dietary goals for the United States. First ed. Washington: U.S. Govt. Print. Off., February 1977.

7. National Advisory Committee on Nutritional Education (NACNE). A discussion paper on proposals for nutritional guidelines for health education in Britain. London: The Health Education Council, 1983.

8. U.S. Department of Health and Human Services and U.S. Department of Agriculture. 2015 – 2020 Dietary Guidelines for Americans. 8th Edition.: Available at http://health.gov/dietaryguidelines/2015/guidelines/. 2015.

9. Harcombe Z, Baker JS, Cooper SM, et al. Evidence from randomised controlled trials did not support the introduction of dietary fat guidelines in 1977 and 1983: a systematic review and meta-analysis. Open Heart 2015;2(1) doi: 10.1136/openhrt-2014-000196.

10. Harcombe Z, Baker JS, DiNicolantonio JJ, Grace F, Davies B. Evidence from randomised controlled trials does not support current dietary fat guidelines: a systematic review and meta-analysis. Open Heart 2016;3(2) doi: 10.1136/openhrt-2016-000409.

11. Dawber TR, Kannel WB. An epidemiologic study of heart disease: the Framingham study. Nutr. Rev. 1958;16(1):1-4.

12. Reaven GM. Banting lecture 1988. Role of insulin resistance in human disease. Diabetes 1988;37(12):1595-607.

13. Joseph R. Kraft. "Diabetes Epidemic & You." Trafford Publishing. (2008).

14. Crofts, C., Zinn, C., Wheldon, M., Schofield, G. 2015. Hyperinsulinemia: A unifying theory of chronic disease?. Diabesity 1(4): 34-43. DOI:10.15562/diabesity.2015.19.

15. Menke A et al. JAMA. 2015 Sep 8;314(10):1021-9. doi: 10.1001/jama.2015.10029. Prevalence of and Trends in Diabetes Among Adults in the United States, 1988-2012.

16. Marja Pyörälä, Heikki Miettinen, Markku Laakso and Kalevi Pyörälä. "Hyperinsulinemia Predicts Coronary Heart Disease Risk in Healthy Middle-aged Men" Circulation. 1998;98:398-404.

Chapter Thirteen

1. Noakes TD. Lore of Running: Human Kinetics Publishers, Champaign, IL 2003.

2. Westman EC, Phinney SD, Volek JS. The New Atkins for a New You. New York: Fireside 2010.

3. Koeslag JH, Noakes TD, Sloan AW. Post-exercise ketosis. *JPhysiol* 1980;301:79-90.

4. Reaven G. Insulin resistance and coronary heart disease in nondiabetic individuals. *Arterioscler Thromb Vasc Biol* 2012;32(8):1754-59.

5. Erpeldinger S, Rehman MB, Berkhout C, et al. Efficacy and safety of insulin in type 2 diabetes: meta-analysis of randomised controlled trials. *BMC endocrine disorders* 2016;16(1):39. doi: 10.1186/s12902-016-0120-z [published Online First: 2016/07/09]

6. Stefansson V. Not by bread alone. New York: The Macmillan Company 1946:1-339.

7. Owen OE, Morgan AP, Kemp HG, et al. Brain metabolism during fasting. *J Clin Invest* 1967;46(10):1589-95.

8. Webster CC, Noakes TD, Chacko SK, et al. Gluconeogenesis during endurance exercise in cyclists habituated to a long-term low carbohydrate high fat diet. *J Physiol* 2016

9. Yeo WK, Carey AL, Burke L, et al. Fat adaptation in well-trained athletes: effects on cell metabolism. *Appl Physiol Nutr Metab* 2011;36(1):12-22. doi: 10.1139/h10-089 [published Online First: 2011/02/18]

10. Institute of Medicine. Dietary Reference Intakes for energy, carbohydrate, fiber, fat, fatty acides, cholesterol, protein and amino acids. Washington DC: National Academies Press 2005:1331.

11. Bowen R. Basic Fermentation Chemistry. *Digestive Physiology of Herbivores* 2010. http://arbl.cvmbs.colostate.edu/hbooks/pathphys/digestion/herbivores/ferment.html.

12. Bowen R. Nutrient absorption and utilization in ruminants. 2009. http://www.vivo.colostate.edu/hbooks/pathphys/digestion/herbivores/rum_absorb.html.

13. Fabbrini E, Higgins PB, Magkos F, et al. Metabolic response to high-carbohydrate and low-carbohydrate meals in a nonhuman primate model. *Am J Physiol Endocrinol Metab* 2013;304(4):E444-E51.

14. Singh VP, Bali A, Singh N, et al. Advanced glycation end products and diabetic complications. *The Korean journal of physiology & pharmacology : official journal of the Korean Physiological Society and the Korean Society of Pharmacology* 2014;18(1):1-14. doi: 10.4196/kjpp.2014.18.1.1 [published Online First: 2014/03/19]

15. Unger RH, Cherrington AD. Glucagonocentric restructuring of diabetes: a pathophysiologic and therapeutic makeover. *J Clin Invest* 2012;122(1):4-12.

16. Hermansen L, Hultman E, Saltin B. Muscle glycogen during prolonged severe exercise. *Acta Physiol Scand* 1967;71(2):129-39.

17. Noakes TD. Fatigue is a Brain-Derived Emotion that Regulates the Exercise Behavior to Ensure the Protection of Whole Body Homeostasis. *Front Physiol* 2012;3:82.

18. NHS. Type 2 diabetes – Steve's story. *NHS Choices* 2016. http://www.nhs.uk/conditions/diabetes-type2/pages/steveredgrave.aspx.

19. Phinney SD, Bistrian BR, Evans WJ, et al. The human metabolic response to chronic ketosis without caloric restriction: preservation of submaximal exercise capability with reduced carbohydrate oxidation. *Metabolism* 1983;32(8):769-76.

20. Burke LM, Hawley JA, Schabort EJ, et al. Carbohydrate loading failed to improve 100-km cycling performance in a placebo-controlled trial. *J Appl Physiol* 2000;88(4):1284-90.

21. Havemann L, West SJ, Goedecke JH, et al. Fat adaptation followed by carbohydrate loading compromises high-intensity sprint performance. *J Appl Physiol* 2006;100(1):194-202.

22. Burke LM, Kiens B. "Fat adaptation" for athletic performance: the nail in the coffin? *Journal of applied physiology (Bethesda, Md : 1985)* 2006;100(1):7-8. doi: 10.1152/japplphysiol.01238.2005 [published Online First: 2005/12/17]

23. Burke LM, Ross ML, Garvican-Lewis LA, et al. Low Carbohydrate, High Fat diet impairs exercise economy and negates the performance benefit from intensified training in elite race walkers. *J Physiol* 2016 doi: 10.1113/jp273230 [published Online First: 2016/12/25]

24. Noakes T, Volek JS, Phinney SD. Low-carbohydrate diets for athletes: what evidence? *Br J Sports Med* 2014;48(14):1077-78.

25. Volek JS, Noakes T, Phinney SD. Rethinking fat as a fuel for endurance exercise. *Eur J Sport Sci* 2015;15(1):13-20.

26. Volek JS, Freidenreich DJ, Saenz C, et al. Metabolic characteristics of keto-adapted ultra-endurance runners. *Metabolism* 2016;65(3):100-10.

27. MacRae HS, Dennis SC, Bosch AN, et al. Effects of training on lactate production and removal during progressive exercise in humans. *J Appl Physiol* 1992;72(5):1649-56.

28. Emhoff CA, Messonnier LA, Horning MA, et al. Direct and indirect lactate oxidation in trained and untrained men. *Journal of applied physiology (Bethesda, Md : 1985)* 2013;115(6):829-38. doi: 10.1152/japplphysiol.00538.2013 [published Online First: 2013/06/22]

29. Jeukendrup A. A step towards personalized sports nutrition: carbohydrate intake during exercise. *Sports Med* 2014;44 Suppl 1:S25-33. doi: 10.1007/s40279-014-0148-z [published Online First: 2014/05/06]

30. Burke LM. Re-Examining High-Fat Diets for Sports Performance: Did We Call the 'Nail in the Coffin' Too Soon? *Sports Med* 2015;45 Suppl 1:S33-49. doi: 10.1007/s40279-015-0393-9 [published Online First: 2015/11/11]

31. McMahon D. After Chris Froome cut back on carbs for more protein, he lost 20 pounds, started winning the Tour de France, and became a millionaire. *Business Insider* 2016; Sports. http://www.businessinsider.com/chris-froome-weight-loss-tour-de-france-2016-7.

32. Genisson U. Romain Bardet un cycliste cétoadapté qui remporte sa première étape du tour de France. *EatFat2BeFit* 2016. www.eatfat2befit.fr/2016/07/romain-bardet-un-cycliste-cetoadapte.html.

33. Brouns F, Saris WH, Stroecken J, et al. Eating, drinking, and cycling. A controlled Tour de France simulation study, Part I. *Int J Sports Med* 1989;10 Suppl 1:S32-40. doi: 10.1055/s-2007-1024952 [published Online First: 1989/05/01]

34. Brouns F, Saris WH, Stroecken J, et al. Eating, drinking, and cycling. A controlled Tour de France simulation study, Part II. Effect of diet manipulation. *Int J Sports Med* 1989;10 Suppl 1:S41-8. doi: 10.1055/s-2007-1024953 [published Online First: 1989/05/01]

35. Schofield G. Understanding how to be the best you can be: Dr Nic Gill, low carb, low sugar and the, All Blacks. *The Science of Human Potential* 2015. https://profgrant.com/2015/11/02/dr-nic-gill-low-carb-low-sugar-and-the-all-blacks/.

36. Smith R. New Head of Nutrition gives Liverpool a taste of Premier League success. *The New York Times* 2016.

37. Hetlelid KJ, Plews DJ, Herold E, et al. Rethinking the role of fat oxidation: substrate utilisation during high-intensity interval training in well-trained and recreationally trained runners. *BMJ open sport & exercise medicine* 2015;1(1):e000047. doi: 10.1136/bmjsem-2015-000047 [published Online First: 2015/08/21]

38. Maffetone P. Eating for endurance. New York, US: David Barmore Productions 1999.

39. Scott D. Twitter feed. July 2016. https://twitter.com/ProfTimNoakes/status/756237621030973441.

40. Polloreno J. Ironman legend Dave Scott shares his nutrition tips. *Triathlete* 2016; 24 Oct. http://www.triathlete.com/2016/10/nutrition/ironman-legend-dave-scott-shares-nutrition-tips_295422.

41. Maffetone P. Eating for endurance: Mark Allen quote. New York, US: David Barmore Productions 1999: p.7.

42. Maffetone P. Eating for endurance: Mike Pigg quote. New York, US: David Barmore Productions 1999: p.9.

43. Maffetone PB, Laursen PB. Athletes: Fit but Unhealthy? *Sports medicine – open* 2016;2(1):24. doi: 10.1186/s40798-016-0048-x [published Online First: 2016/10/18]

44. Maffetone P. Case study: Reductions in training load and dietary carbohydrates help restore health and improve performance in an Ironman triathlete. 2016. https://philmaffetone.com/case-study-reductions-training-load-dietary-carbohydrates-help-restore-health-improve-performance-ironman-triathlete/.

45. Noakes T. Time to quit that marathon running? Not quite yet! *Basic Res Cardiol* 2014;109(1):395.

46. Möhlenkamp S, Lehmann N, Breuckmann F, et al. Running: the risk of coronary events : Prevalence and prognostic relevance of coronary atherosclerosis in marathon runners. *Eur Heart J* 2008;29(15):1903-10. doi: 10.1093/eurheartj/ehn163 [published Online First: 2008/04/23]

47. Noakes TD, Creed S-A, Proudfoot J, et al. The Real Meal Revolution. 2nd edition ed. Cape Town: Quivertree Publications 2013:1-298.

48. Cryer PE, White NH, Santiago JV. The relevance of glucose counterregulatory systems to patients with insulin-dependent diabetes mellitus. *Endocrine reviews* 1986;7(2):131-9. doi: 10.1210/edrv-7-2-131 [published Online First: 1986/05/01]

49. Greenhalgh PM. Competitive sport and the insulin-dependent diabetic patient. *Postgrad Med J* 1990;66(780):803-6. [published Online First: 1990/10/01]

50. Berger M, Hagg S, Ruderman NB. Glucose metabolism in perfused skeletal muscle. Interaction of insulin and exercise on glucose uptake. *Biochem J* 1975;146(1):231-8. [published Online First: 1975/01/01]

51. Galbo H. Hormonal and metabolic adaptation to exercise. Stuttgart, New York: Georg Thieme 1983.

Chapter Fourteen

1. Hereafter, "Type 2 Diabetes" will simply be referred to as "diabetes."

2. http://www.zoeharcombe.com/2015/10/jennifer-elliott-vs-dietitians-association-of-australia/

3. http://www.scirp.org/journal/PaperInformation.aspx?PaperID=50455

4. https://daa.asn.au/voice-of-daa/public-statements/

5. http://www.babyboomersandbellies.com/blog/2015/08/my-case-with-daa-revisited-or-revisiting-my-case-with-daa-or-daa-revisited/

6. https://www.scribd.com/document/348345200/AHPRA-Sept-7-2016

7. http://www.nofructose.com/gary-fettke/

8. https://www.ahpra.gov.au/News/2016-11-16-media-statement.aspx

9. https://www.scribd.com/document/348414603/APHRA-caution-of-Fettke

10. http://foodmed.net/2016/11/30/gary-fettke-kangaroo-court-australia-lchf-part-2/

11. http://www.aph.gov.au/Parliamentary_Business/Committees/Senate/Community_Affairs/ComplaintsMechanism/Report , Chapter 6.

12. http://www.mensfitness.com/nutrition/what-to-eat/truth-behind-worlds-most-cutting-edge-fat-burning-performance-meal-plan-keto

13. https://www.outsideonline.com/2140271/silencing-low-carb-rebel

14. http://www.thenoakesfoundation.org/prof-noakes

15. https://www.amazon.com/New-Atkins-You-Ultimate-Shedding/dp/1439190275

16. http://www.thebigfatfix.com

17. Personal observation during a visit to Cape Town in October 2016, to testify for the defense in the Noakes hearing.

18. Interview with Tim Noakes, October 2016.

19. http://www.zoeharcombe.com/2016/10/the-hpcsa-vs-professor-noakes/

20. http://foodmed.net/2016/11/04/caryn-zinn-to-parents-dont-feed-cereals-to-babies/

21. http://foodmed.net/2016/10/26/nina-teicholz-low-fat-diets-can-kill/
http://foodmed.net/2016/10/26/noakes-trial-nina-teicholz-explodes-fat-bombs/

22. http://foodmed.net/2016/04/13/noakes-low-fat-causes-heart-disease-lchf-banting/
http://foodmed.net/2016/02/21/noakes-sa-dietary-guidelines-misguidelines-lchf-banting-hpcsa/

23. http://journals.plos.org/plosone/article/related?id=10.1371/journal.pone.0100652

24. http://www.zoeharcombe.com/2017/04/prof-noakes-stellenbosch-the-exchanges/

25. http://www.samj.org.za/index.php/samj/article/view/11605/7753

26. http://www.zoeharcombe.com/2017/04/prof-noakes-stellenbosch-the-exchanges/

27. https://www.scribd.com/document/348273228/Tim-Noakes-Judgement-HPCSA-Final

28. http://www.news24.com/Video/SouthAfrica/News/watch-tim-noakes-elated-with-not-guilty-verdict-20170421

29. http://www.health24.com/Diet-and-nutrition/Nutrition-basics/noakes-slams-hpcsa-witch-hunt-as-body-appeals-not-guilty-ruling-20170512

30. Teicholz, N. *The Big Fat Surprise* (Simon & Schuster 2014), p. 134.

31. Ibid, pp. 62-63.

32. Ibid, p. 245.

33. Ibid, p. 247.

34. https://www.wsj.com/articles/the-questionable-link-between-saturated-fat-and-heart-disease-1399070926

35. http://www.huffingtonpost.com/david-katz-md/sugar-and-saturated-fat-f_b_8227088.html

36. http://www.huffingtonpost.com/david-katz-md/national-nutrition-policy_b_8380658.html

37. https://www.theguardian.com/society/2016/apr/07/the-sugar-conspiracy-robert-lustig-john-yudkin

38. http://www.huffingtonpost.com/david-katz-md/diet-and-nutrition_b_5266165.html

39. Teicholz, N., op. cit., p. 126.

40. Ibid, pp. 125-126.

41. http://thehill.com/blogs/congress-blog/healthcare/257353-coalition-is-full-of-baloney-on-nutrition-guidelines

42. http://www.bmj.com/content/351/bmj.h4962

43. http://www.bmj.com/content/351/bmj.h4962/rr

44. http://www.bmj.com/content/351/bmj.h4962/rr-1

45. http://www.bmj.com/content/351/bmj.h4962/rr-32

46. https://www.theguardian.com/society/2016/apr/07/the-sugar-conspiracy-robert-lustig-john-yudkin

https://www.scribd.com/lists/15280507/11-5-15-retraction-request-sent-to-BMJ-by-CSPI

47. http://www.bmj.com/company/wp-content/uploads/2016/12/the-bmj-US-dietary-correction.pdf

48. http://www.the-sidebar.com/2016/03/craven-cave-in-how-journalistauthor.html
http://www.the-sidebar.com/2016/05/did-usda-executive-angela-tagtow.html
http://www.politico.com/tipsheets/morning-agriculture/2016/03/teicholz-disinvited-from-food-policy-panel-stabenow-grassley-let-usda-fda-review-syngenta-merger-fda-to-release-food-safety-tests-on-cucumbers-213410

49. http://www.spiked-online.com/newsite/article/fat-chance-of-a-debate-meet-the-foodie-censors/18249#.WRikfRiZM0r

50. http://www.ipetitions.com/petition/reinstate-teicholz-on-food-policy-panel

51. https://therussells.crossfit.com/2017/01/05/big-food-vs-tim-noakes-the-final-crusade/

52. https://therussells.crossfit.com/2016/09/26/david-katz-junk-foods-slyest-defender/

Glossary

ADSA	Association for Dietetics in South Africa
AHA	American Heart Association
AHPRA	Australian Health Practitioners Regulatory Authority
AUT	Auckland University of Technology
BMI	Body Mass Index
BMJ	British Medical Journal
CDC	(US) The Centers for Disease Control and Prevention
CGM	Continuous Glucose Monitors
CHCD	Chronic Non-Communicable Diseases
CHD	Coronary Heart Disease
CSPI	Center for Science in the Public Interest
CVD	Cardiovascular Disease
DAA	Dietitians Association of Australia
DAFNE	Dose Adjustment For Normal Eating
DART	Diet and Reinfarction Trial
DGAC	Dietary Guidelines Advisory Committee
DGA	Dietary Guidelines for Americans
DNL	De Novo Lipogenesis
DUI	Driving Under Influence
EBSA	Eat Better South Africa (one of The Noakes Foundation initiatives)
EGP	Endogenous Glucose Production
FFA	Free Fatty Acids
GGT	Gamma-Glutamyl Transferase – a liver enzyme
GI	Glycemic Index
GL	Glycemic Load

HbA1c	Glycated haemoglobin
HDL	High Density Lipoprotein (HDL-C refers to the cholesterol part of HDL)
HPCSA	Health Professions Council of South Africa
IBS	Irritable Bowel Syndrome
IFG	Impaired Fasting Glucose
IGT	Impaired Glucose Tolerance
LCHF	Low Carbohydrate High Fat (sometimes called Low Carbohydrate Healthy Fat)
LFHC	Low Fat High Carbohydrate (or HCLF – High Carb Low Fat)
LDL	Low Density Lipoprotein (LDL-C refers to the cholesterol part of LDL)
MODY	Maturity Onset Diabetes of the Young
NAFLD	Non Alcoholic Fatty Liver Disease
NDPP	National Diabetes Prevention Programme
NFA	(Sweden) National Food Administration
NHS	(UK) National Health Service
NICE	(UK) National Institute for Care and Health Excellence
OGTT	Oral Glucose Tolerance Test
PCSK9	Proprotein Convertase Subtilisin/Kexin type 9 inhibitors – a cholesterol lowering drug
RCT	Randomised Controlled Trial
STARS	St Thomas's Atherosclerosis Regression Study
T1DM	Type 1 Diabetes Mellitus
T2DM	Type 2 Diabetes Mellitus
TC	Total Cholesterol
VFAs	Volatile Fatty Acids
VLDL	Very Low Density Lipoprotein
WHO	World Health Organization

Index

301

protein 49, 67, 71, 73, 82, 89, 101, 104, 118, 123, 150, 151, 152, 153, 170, 188, 195, 198, 206, 226, 233, 237, 240, 242, 243, 244, 248, 257, 258, 259, 291, 292;

Q

Quality and Outcome Framework 175;

R

rabbits 189, 209;
Randomized controlled trials (RCTs) 66, 286;
Reaven, Dr Jerry 42, 43, 219, 220, 221, 225, 290, 291;
Reaven's syndrome 43;
Redgrave, Sir Steven 256;
remission 7, 17, 22, 69, 71, 72, 73, 74, 75, 79, 80, 81, 83, 90, 168;
Research Committee low-fat diet 193;
rugby 230, 254, 255;
ruminants 243, 291;

S

saturated fat 24, 47, 104, 116, 118, 119, 120, 123, 144, 147, 151, 188, 190, 191, 192, 194, 196, 197, 199, 200, 201, 204, 209, 211, 212, 213, 214, 215, 225, 274, 286, 288, 289;
Schofield, Professor Grant 24, 144, 150, 280, 281, 290, 293;
scrotal cancer 187, 188;
Seven Countries Study 191, 192, 194, 195, 211, 212, 214, 219;
Skeaff and Miller 195;
smallpox 57;
smoking 72, 75, 81, 84, 210, 216, 224, 226;
South Africa 7, 8, 9, 10, 20, 21, 22, 26, 143, 232, 263, 264, 265;
stress 21, 33, 36, 55, 76, 84, 109, 152, 175, 176, 216, 222, 226, 270;
St Thomas' Atherosclerosis Regression Study (STARS) 192, 284;
sulphonylureas 46;

Swedish National Board of Health 23, 116;
Syndrome X 43, 219;
systematic review 86, 173, 191, 192, 199, 277, 278, 280, 283, 284, 286, 289, 290;

T

Taubes, Gary 280;
Taylor, Professor Roy 134, 173, 179, 282;
Teicholz, Nina 6, 20, 261, 280, 295;
The Family Food Survey 201, 289;
thirst 15, 54, 70, 71, 72, 82, 147, 264;
Time Magazine 195, 212, 225, 286;
Tour de France 230, 254, 292, 293;
toxic 8, 61, 62, 63, 65, 66, 70, 73, 74, 75, 78, 79, 217, 222, 224, 248;
Triathlon 230, 252, 253, 255, 256, 257, 258;

U

Unwin, Dr David 6, 24, 139, 167, 180, 282;
urine 37, 38, 39, 46, 78;

V

vaccines 57;
VLDL 43, 44, 46, 210;
Volek, Professor Jeff 231, 252, 291, 292;

W

Walker, Clare 48, 49, 50;
Wellington, Dr Neville 6, 24, 159, 165;
Westman, Dr Eric 231, 232, 291;
Whitington, Jen 5, 23, 127, 128, 135;
World Health Organisation 278;

Y

Yerushalmy and Hilleboe 190;

Z

Zinn, Dr Caryn 6, 20, 24, 143, 153, 157, 265, 280, 281, 290;